The Biopolitics of Embryos
and Alphabets

The Biopolitics of Embryos and Alphabets

A Reproductive History of the Nonhuman

RUTH A. MILLER

OXFORD
UNIVERSITY PRESS

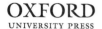

Oxford University Press is a department of the University of Oxford. It furthers
the University's objective of excellence in research, scholarship, and education
by publishing worldwide. Oxford is a registered trade mark of Oxford University
Press in the UK and certain other countries.

Published in the United States of America by Oxford University Press
190 Madison Avenue, New York, NY 10016, United States of America.

Library of Congress Cataloging-in-Publication Data
Names: Miller, Ruth Austin, 1975–
Title: The biopolitics of embryos and alphabets : a reproductive history of
the nonhuman / Ruth A. Miller.
Description: New York, NY : Oxford University Press, [2017] |
Includes bibliographical references and index.
Identifiers: LCCN 2016059040 | ISBN 9780190638351 (hardcover : alk. paper) |
ISBN 9780190638368 (pbk. : alk. paper) | ISBN 9780190638382 (epub) |
ISBN 9780190638375 (updf)
Subjects: LCSH: Bioethics. | Biology—Political aspects. | Biology—Social aspects. |
Reproduction—Political aspects. | Reproduction—Social aspects. |
Reproductive rights. | Sociobiology.
Classification: LCC QH332.M55 2017 | DDC 174.2—dc23
LC record available at https://lccn.loc.gov/2016059040

1 3 5 7 9 8 6 4 2
Paperback printed by Webcom, Inc., Canada
Hardback printed by Bridgeport National Bindery, Inc., United States of America

For my mother, Betsy, and her motorcycle
(September 22, 1938, to March 6, 2015)

CONTENTS

The Biopolitics of Embryos
and Alphabets

Introduction

L ook through the door of the model room, and see box after box, row after row, of magnified and miniature, opaque and transparent, sculptures and carvings of human embryos. Some bulge with detailed surfaces. Some are cut through with faceted interiors. Sturdy tables support polished glass and plastic containers. But the model room is not all there is to see. Don't forget the preserved embryos themselves—cut thinner and thinner into nearly 200,000 serial sections.[1] There could have been more—a serial collection, by definition, never ends,[2] and there is nothing more satisfying than collecting and compiling ever more delicate, molecule-thin slices, strands, and shards of matter.[3] And then displaying them. The Blechschmidt Collection at the University of Göttingen does it well. But the Blechschmidt Collection is certainly not unique.

Consider the Carnegie Collection. Its curators acquired many of the Blechschmidt sections, assigning them Carnegie Nos. 10315-10434,[4] before eventually returning them to the University of Göttingen at the end of the twentieth century—like colonial archaeological detritus taken to museums at the metropole and then sheepishly returned one hundred fifty years later, with apologies. The Carnegie Collection may mourn its now empty files and containers. But there is much still to celebrate—for example, its thousands of slides, its hundreds of whole embryos, its images, mounts, drawings, and specimens "from 3 mm to 310 mm," and its thousands of "serial sections of normal human embryo development."[5] Or perhaps the Hubrecht Collection at the Leibniz Institute for Research on Evolution and Biodiversity is more appealing.[6] Or the Kyoto Collection? It preserves, among other items, "129 embryos with polydactyly in 36,380 human conceptuses obtained through induced abortion during the period from 1962 to 1974."[7]

Or is it perhaps the case that flourishing, organic, ever-increasing—even if only via thinner and thinner slices, microscopic, and then inevitably digital—embryo collections in *stasis* do not seem sufficiently alive? The US state of Louisiana can fix that. Disposing of fertilized human reproductive material being illegal, the state is facing a storage problem. The shiny glass and plastic containers of Blechschmidt's models are a drop in the reproductive bucket compared to the endless receptacles full of frozen, viable, yet not quite desirable, embryos kept under "guardianship" in Louisiana's facilities.[8] The display may not be as felicitous as the displays developed by careful curators in Göttingen, Washington, DC, Utrecht, and Kyoto, but the message—if unintended—is unexpectedly complementary. Look at the reproduction. Watch the growth. Consider the creeping monstrosity that is not the unitary fetus—not even the abnormal unitary fetus with its discrete, if problem, body—but rather the pieces, slices, and bits of multiple, multiplying fetuses, grouped into undifferentiated masses, seeping incrementally into every space, spreading out across one room, many rooms, buildings, institutes, urban grids, rural storage areas.

It's an odd curatorial invitation, if you think about it. Not ethically odd—although if it does strike thus, that's not necessarily a problem. But politically, intellectually, and perhaps aesthetically odd. Why force reproductive growth—modeled in plasticine or otherwise—into conversation with legal and scientific rationality, and then in turn with nostalgia? Nostalgia, after all, is clearly compelling this antiquarian fixation on completing serial sets of sliced up specimens—just as much as nostalgia is motivating Louisiana's melancholy, arrested, non-developing matter: this matter that is always looking back to an initiating moment that, nostalgically, never quite makes good on its promised future.[9] What could reproductive growth, law, science, and something as squeamish as nostalgia ever have to do with one another? Or, more to the point, what could they say to one another under these circumstances that so drastically and almost parodically obliterate the embodied human subject, the person who is ordinarily at stake in the law of reproduction, in philosophies of rational interaction with the world, and in the disengaged ecstasy or despair of nostalgia? Did I mention that the Carnegie Collection also throws together pig, mouse, and "other" embryonic material in its displays—just to mix things up?

The answer to these questions, provisionally, is that nostalgia, nonhuman (or obliterated human) reproduction, and politics have everything to do with one another. The curators—and Louisiana's storage facilities—do, it turns out, have something of a point. These simultaneously nostalgic and hyper-rational displays of disembodied reproduction, of replication that is also growth and enlargement, are displays of a particular type of politics, of a particular meditation on mass democracy. On view, for everyone to witness, is a politics of life, unbounded, in its most pristine form. Gobbling up and squirting out all sorts of stuff that, again provisionally, codes as human—embryos, fetuses, slides, statistics, genetic material, law, rationality, positivist certainty, and incurable melancholy—these displays mutter to anyone willing to listen that when life becomes the object of science, politics, and law, the human, or human genetic code at the very least, runs up against a glitch. The embodied, thinking, bounded, self-conscious human becomes a farce, a series of up to 200,000 slices of matter, distributed across a thousand, so they say, platforms, mediums, and ok, plateaus.[10]

But, you remark, we already know this. These sliced up embryos are an extreme example of it, but the history of biopolitics—not to mention the seemingly perpetual politics of biopolitics—along with its occasional posthuman corollary, played out, interminably, in the scholarship of the

1990s and early 2000s. The fact that Michel Foucault, in his 1975–1976 lectures, "Society Must be Defended," and in the first volume of his *History of Sexuality*, floated this term, "biopolitics"—positing that in the eighteenth century the sovereign right over life shifted from the right to kill to the right to manage and prolong biological existence[11]—has been well and truly commemorated. Likewise, the implications of this modern democratic collision of biology, on the one hand, and politics, on the other— the implications of a flourishing modern rhetoric of "life" as a biological or environmental, rather than legal or linguistic, problem[12]—gave rise to countless scholarly conferences a good twenty years ago. Obviously the human, the person, is drawn up short (or stretched out long), hacked into pieces, distributed catastrophically across equally countless statistical apparatuses when the politics of thought, of sovereignty, of rights, of speech, and of liberty gives way to the politics of reproduction, of dirt, of matter, and of freakishly flourishing, growing, spreading, living life.[13] Obviously, the liberal fantasy of a rational, thinking, speaking subject of politics—the discrete, bounded person, with property, even, in his (and occasionally, if grudgingly, her) body—is replaced by the Blechschmidt Collection's fantasy of ever thinner slices of embryonic material, when birth and death become a problem for the undifferentiated population or nation rather than a problem of the individual citizen.[14] That has been done. Academics, at least, were quite glad to see the tail end of it.[15]

Equally well done is the ethical response to this work—necessary if frequently underappreciated: the well taken point that losing the human and focusing on the vitality, though catastrophic in the "ending and overturning" sense of the term, is not the horror that it might seem to be.[16] On the contrary, a politics of, specifically, unbounded, nonhuman, noncognitive life, reproduction, and replication has a lot to recommend it.[17] If nothing else, empirically, it seems a more effective framework of inquiry when it comes to addressing key and bewildering plot points in modern, mass democratic history than the works that slavishly seek to capture and frame the forever missing Person. At most, this now passé scholarship prevents an increasingly perplexing (and no doubt perplexed) array of nonhuman things, systems, assemblages, aggregates, forces, energies, and stuff—everything from trees to the passage of time—from being squashed into the far more perilous procrustean bed of honorary human status, complete with humanesque rights. Let's grant climate change the right to property! The moon's gravitational pull the right to education! If we're just tolerant and inclusive enough, liberal democracy can solve anything!

Anyhow, the point here, once more, is that the history of biopolitics, with its posthuman implications, has already been written. Ad infinitum. And the ethics of biopolitics perhaps just needs to be quiet. We know the stakes: there is a tension between liberal democracy with its focus, broadly, on thought, and biopolitics (or biopolitical democracy) with its focus, broadly, on life. Responses at the two extremes of the spectrum have included, on the one hand, sending out the superheroes to rescue the human from his (yes, that's deliberate) appalling, sickening, ghoulish Life,[18] and, on the other hand, celebrating the death (or early term abortion) of the human who, in any case, didn't particularly enjoy his life to begin with.[19]

There have been more measured responses as well. Thought has been redefined as a not purely human affair—meekly welcome in the nonhuman, not quite human, inhuman politics of life—and thus liberal democracy and biopolitical democracy have begun to blend and bleed together (again).[20] Life, likewise, has crept inexorably from minds to subjects to bodies to systems to assemblages to matter to fascinating sets of objects that caper around material, organic, inorganic, and digital pastures and deserts, shocking not just the bourgeoisie with their weirdly, too human pluckiness. And biopolitical democratic engagement, in turn, in this way, becomes not so much something to fear or to advocate as something to observe, bemused from the smooth, edge-less surfaces of John Dewey's public sphere.[21] Both human-centripetal and human-centrifugal takes on biopolitics—as well as biopolitics in conversation with liberal politics—have received, in short, their due.

But—and there's that familiar sinking feeling—let's do it again. Here's why. (Although first, an assurance—what follows is short, sketchy, schematic, and woefully insufficient; I promise more detail in the next chapter.) The classic split or rift—as much as it has been healed, pasted over, or taped together—between biopolitics and liberal politics has been a split between a politics that privileges reproduction (or, to include the capering objects and their digital compatriots, replication) and a politics that privileges cognitive or affective thought. Liberal politics celebrates cognition and affect; biopolitics celebrates reproducing matter.[22] Never the twain shall meet.[23]

Let's bracket, for the moment, the shocking revelations of democracies of life that have secretly and spectacularly dealt in death.[24] Let's pay no attention, that is to say, to Giorgio Agamben's now likewise passé point that the genocidal concentration camp, rather than the city, has always been the most logical space of life-obsessed (biopolitical) democratic engagement.[25] And let's similarly ignore the democracies of thought that have unapologetically eradicated the merest possibility of thinking, shunting all cognition (not to mention affect) into the narrow, confined corridors of rational dialogue.[26] Forget the work of feminist legal theorists who have noted what Wendy Brown has described as "the regulatory potential in speaking ourselves, its capacity to bind rather than emancipate us,"[27] or what Marianne Constable has posited as the "possibilities of justice that lie in silence," given the claustrophobic quality of even the most liberated speech.[28] The internal contradictions within democracies that celebrate *either* life *or* speech are less important, at least here, than the apparent, and more fundamental, split underlying these (nonetheless valid) critiques: the politics of cognitive or affective thought and the politics of reproductive or replicating life do not get along, even when they fail to function according to their own terms. We either have to choose our side—Descartes damning us all to an impossible set of alternatives— or redefine our terms (maybe Cartesian matter and Cartesian thought are not the hellishly dichotomous categories we have all assumed them to be).[29] Reproducing matter (or information[30]) and thinking matter (or information) cannot occupy the same political place.

Unless—and here is the punchline of this introduction to the Introduction—the reproducing matter and the thinking matter are taking a holiday in Göttingen and viewing the Blechschmidt collection. Or perusing the Carnegie embryos. Or touring Utrecht's lantern slides or

Kyoto's mid-century specimens. Or, obviously, breaking into Louisiana's storage facilities and peeking into the well-guarded containers from a nicely concealed cooling duct. Remember, though: in all of these vacation spots, reproduction, growth, replication, and flourishing have slammed inexorably not just into rationality, not just into law and politics, but also into melancholy and nostalgia. Nostalgia rescues unbounded matter from the impossible opposition between life and thought, between liberal and biopolitical democratic engagement. Nostalgia—that disreputable, sentimental yearning for a unitary, imaginary past that promises, in turn, a flat, disengaged, and impossible future, or that irresponsible transformation of complex space into pure sensation and memory, or even that decontextualization of event or moment in the name of impression or apprehension[31]—is the mode of engagement with the world that allows thought and life to coexist, productively, within democratic politics. That is the thesis of this book.

Call what follows, therefore, a nonhuman biopolitics of nostalgia; or perhaps, a melancholy history of nonhuman biopolitical thought. But do not misunderstand: there is nothing diffuse about these terms. The arguments driving this book are insistent, hell-bent, and unrelenting: First, there has never been a tension between the reproductive life of biopolitics, on the one hand, and the cognitive or affective thought of liberalism, on the other. On the contrary, reproduction has always been identical to thought in modern mass democracy. Second, more pointedly, narrowly, sharply, reproduction has been identical not just to thought, but to nostalgia—a type of thought or memory ordinarily associated only with human subjectivity. The most effective way to recognize the total simultaneity of reproductive life and nostalgic thought, however, is to take the nonhuman—the radically nonhuman (think slime mold rather than puppies)—as a political norm.[32] What you will find here, therefore, in this melancholy nonhuman history of biopolitical nostalgic thought, is a story of nonhuman reproduction as nonhuman nostalgia in modern mass democracy.

No matter how emphatic the italics in the previous paragraph, however, there are some obstacles already bloodying our sliding fingertips, as we lose ever more traction, pulling ourselves to the first ledge in this climb. In a spirit of optimism, though, call these obstacles "implications" to be explored, over the following chapters. Most notable of these complicated implications, for example, is the scent in the air—the hint of healthy scholarly bloodlust—that the posthuman, like "biopolitics," is in need of a good trend-setting (the term is usually "field transforming") slaughter.[33] People are getting bored and thus violent. Animal studies was fine.[34] The environment needed some critical attention. Bacteria, microbes, and algorithms were just successful and terrifying enough to be actant-entertaining. We also got to cite a lot of speculative fiction from the 1980s when we got cozy with that matter. But really, what's wrong with anthropocentrism? People in the know have made it clear that the nonhuman is at this point, at best, an embarrassment. There's a rumor that Slavoj Žižek is writing a book.[35]

Nonetheless, at the risk of setting up for merciless mockery all of the innocent information and guiltless slime that will smear themselves across the (likely digital) pages of this book, there will be much apologizing for posthuman studies throughout the following pages. In addition to chapter 1—an extended review of feminist theories of nonhuman politics, life, and reproduction—a healthy dose of empirical historical evidence will ground, in later chapters, heavily, stodgily, this compulsive return to the posthuman. *Historically*, these pages, jabbing an insistent finger in the air, will insist, the politics of reproductive life has taken nonhuman assemblages as its norm. *Historically*, reproduction, as a political activity, has dissolved into thought, memory, and nostalgia. And *historically*, the nostalgia of unbounded, nonhuman things, growths, and accumulations, reproducing and replicating themselves, has been the basis of mass democratic engagement.

Hysterically insisting on the value of nonhuman frameworks of analysis, despite the march of academic progress, and despite the half-smug, half-mortified smirks of graduate students, is, thus, a good faith move. Give the material from the archives and libraries a chance. Odd as it may be—with variations on the theme of embryonic goo standing in for nostalgic reproducing slime, and obliterated Turkish alphabets alongside, quietly, secretly, stashes of American metadata (the data of hordes alongside the hoards of data—data on horses?) standing in for nostalgic replicating information—it tells a compelling story. There is a case to be made for, first, mass democracy as a classically nonhuman affair and second, nostalgic, unbounded, likewise nonhuman reproduction as the political activity that makes this democracy happen. Watch and see.

Second obstacle—more stubbed toe than bloodied fingers: biopolitics came to no good in the academy in large part because it seemed not to solve anything. The posthuman is facing the same sad fate. What actually does reveling in the potential politics of the creepy growth of a sadistic squash vine, strangling the life out of less aggressive assemblages, as it flourishes across some hapless Darwinian heath, do for us? Yes, those spiral tendrils are pretty. And true, it can help to explain the course of historical mass democracy as a history of life writ large. But what can it do for us *now*? In the old tradition of shifted paradigms,[36] a quick revel in the assemblage can, broadly, still open up new avenues of inquiry and new ethical systems. So many frightening, fascinating monstrosities in the world—so many nonhuman, subhuman, utterly inhuman threats to democracy, so many hoards upon hordes making inroads into our fragile mode of governance—it makes sense, if not to wrap our minds around them, at least to let them seep into the unprotected bits that we aren't really using. We have to know them to fight them.

But perhaps, against this militaristic inclination, these aggregates and accumulations are not threats. That doesn't make them—or their mode of political engagement—any less worth foregrounding. Rethinking democracy as a nonhuman affair, and nonhuman replication as a democratic act, helps shove these accumulations of information and things in that direction. This finger-jabbing insistence on ignoring the menace in order to explore nonhuman political potential, however, is nonetheless still not as easy as it might seem to be. Indeed, as much as the embryonic slices of the Blechschmidt collection may provoke a chill, albeit once removed in history, and inappropriate in any case because it's all in the name of science, other reproductive slime is far more serious.

The embryonic goo that is the human clone, for example, is legally and literally, at least in liberal Europe, the very worst thing in the world—on par with genocide (and piracy).[37] The reproductive gunk that accidentally slips into the trash is ethically identical to the worst mid-century super villain.[38] Everyone knows that data mines undermine democratic process, belching up stores of information over which ghoulish surveillance states gloat.[39] And although the Turkish Republic's decision to throw over its pre-existing alphabet in the name of early-twentieth-century racial progress is not a chapter in global politics that gets as much play as enslaved (by definition[40]) clones, recycled reproductive matter, and rampant data collection, thoughtful fourteen-year-olds with a copy of *1984* in their pockets all know perfectly well that it is a short, sweet step from policing speech and writing to torturing poor Winston into forgetting the self-evident rules of arithmetic. When in 1928, Turkey's parliament legislated a nationwide shift from Arabic to Latin alphabetic characters, that is to say—thereby rendering its reading and writing population illiterate in a single legal-political stroke—this move toward what Republican nationalists liked to call Western Civilization, with its Latin rather than Arabic characters, smacked as much of what those fourteen-year-olds would, in turn, call thought control as it did of a glorious partnership with Turkey's European confederates.

Or, for that matter, consider nostalgia. Nostalgia—a bit of pseudo-psychological flotsam jettisoned from the nineteenth-century sanatorium with its electricity and cold baths, a nasty neologism fashioned from *algia*, pain, and *nostos*, longing for home[41]—has been re-energized and set wafting jauntily over the waves of politics and psychology as one of the true evils facing the responsible, engaged self. Nostalgia is bad.[42] It saps the energies—if no longer the psychic energies, then at least their proper political counterparts—by making a mockery of the here and the now, of that point in linear time at which something can, and must, be done.[43] Intriguingly, scholars of nostalgia have been falling all over themselves to recuperate the concept in a less livid way (more on that in chapter 2). Nostalgia, if kept at an appropriate distance, they write, can be bracingly humanizing. It can quell the quivering fear induced by the politics of that nutty squash vine—by the democracy of those alienating technological[44] growths, accumulations, and hoards.[45] Conventional scholarly wisdom, however, remains relatively united: nostalgia is on par with slavery and surveillance as a political ill to cure.

And in any case, here, the restoration and resuscitation of nostalgia involves not breathing the oxygen of human life back into its decrepit, pre-Freudian, neurasthenic body, but giving it a few hints from the realm of cyano-bacteria. Nostalgia, like reproduction and life, works, if it does work, politically because it is *not* human. It enjoys its noxious fumes. And if the most politically relevant mode of reproduction, replication, and flourishing—that enjoyed, eccentrically and ecstatically, by accumulations of slime and data that transgress nothing because they have no feet to take the necessary steps—can indeed be linked to nostalgia, then nostalgia is a key contemporary rediscovery; just not the one it may seem to be. Take nostalgia seriously. Its play across unbounded, nonhuman accumulations has historically produced, secreted, excreted, and defecated democratic engagement (at least, so will say the jabbing finger); and its ongoing creep and calcification form the only touchstones by which to evaluate contemporary problems in policy.

Or, more generally, watch the following three defenses unfold over the next chapters: a defense, first, of the pure politics of posthuman reproduction; a defense, second, of nonhuman, never human democracy; and a defense, third, of the nostalgia of embryos and alphabets. Modern governance, these pages assert, would fall apart without them. Indeed, it is the fact that these nonhuman assemblages are capable of existing nostalgically in a way that purely human political subjects are not that grants them their political force. When the embryo, for example, becomes an environment in which senses and memories are physically, nostalgically embedded over time—and in which these memories are repeatedly detached and recontextualized in the name of reproductive growth—an arena unfolds in which thought and reproduction are equally viable political activities. The embryo, because of its nostalgia—because of its translation or flattening of spaces, environments, and times into half-remembered sensitivities— offers up hope, in a way that less nostalgic figures do not, for a democratic politics of thinking life. Similarly, the exterminated alphabet, as a reproductive or replicating environment, distributes sentimental memories throughout space and time—transforming spaces and times into impressionistic memories. Once it is replaced by the new alphabet and no longer a vehicle of dialogue or speech, that is to say, the dead alphabet, like the embryo, because of its nostalgia, allows for the reintroduction of political life to political thought. This defense of nostalgia—of nonhuman nostalgia—therefore is an ardent one: nonhuman nostalgia of this sort serves as a unique platform for political hope.

What follows, then, are four chapters that make a political case for the nostalgia of, narrowly, embryos and alphabets.[46] Two of these chapters are short and two are long—although packed into the short ones are the themes and arguments that (before the archival dump engulfs the long chapters) will, if not convince you of, at least, hopefully, intrigue you into considering, the possibility that nonhuman political life is a variation on nonhuman nostalgia. These short chapters will posit, first, that when nonhuman assemblages such as embryos and exterminated alphabets live and reproduce, they transform—just as slime mold does—environments and spaces into physical memory and sensation. Second, these chapters will suggest that the transformation of environment or space into memory or sensation, and that the decontextualization and recontextualization of space, sense, and matter undertaken by these assemblages, is, by definition (see chapter 2), a mode of nostalgia. And third, these chapters will sketch the contours of the broader claim driving the longer chapters that this nostalgic life and reproduction are not only political—just as human reproduction is political—but also politically productive, opening up a framework, once more, for life and thought to complement, rather than compete with, one another, even as democracy continues to limp along.

More specifically, the first of these short chapters presents key, evocative moments in various feminist theories of biopolitics. Here are, first, a few indications of the political force of nonhuman life, reproduction, and thought, both historically and in the here and now, and second, a set of proofs that this life, reproduction, and thought are so intermingled as to be, chemically, aesthetically, and ethically, the same thing: when nonhuman biopolitics becomes thinkable as a democratic norm, the simultaneity of the reproduction of life and the contemplation of life likewise become a jingle impossible to expel from our collective head. Shift the framework, re-shuffle the Bakelite viewmaster, and they are always, insistently, the same thing.

The second short chapter is a literature review of a completely different—politically, methodologically, ethically, aesthetically—set of texts: in this case, those dealing with the history, literature, and theory of nostalgia. Nostalgia has become a topic of mild, increasing interest—nothing close to, say, vampires in the late 1990s, but respectable—over the past few decades. Cynically extracting the strands of this scholarship that are relevant to the theories trotted out here, this chapter invites across the threshold several claims: first, that nostalgia in fact easily lends itself to nonhuman manifestations, second, that this nonhuman nostalgia is not as ethically questionable as commentators on nostalgia writ large have hinted it is, and third, that nonhuman nostalgia may very well therefore be the sticky paste that holds biopolitics—as a proper and affirmative mode of contemporary mass democratic engagement—together. In this chapter, the literature on feminist biopolitics and the literature on nostalgia as illness and experience suck one another dry, and in the process the two give rise to an altogether different, amalgamated interpretation of political life and thought, one with potentially quite a bit more undead staying power.

The second two major chapters, longer, sometimes plodding, are gratuitous collections of academic curios. They are hoards and heaps of examples from the political history of, first, embryos and, second, alphabets. Each thus shoots at the reader, in an archivally overwhelming way, moment after moment, passage after passage, experience after experience, each piled up into a mountain of tangentially connected examples that will indicate, by their sheer quantity and enormity, that slime (embryos) and data (alphabets) are, indeed, biopolitically alive—are, indeed, biopolitically reproductive, and are likewise productive, in their fecundity, of nonhuman nostalgia. These two case studies are also useful in a more targeted way because they demonstrate the effectiveness of feminist theoretical methods. Embryonic matter has received quite a bit of attention from scholars of gender and sexuality studies. So too have speech and language. Script—alphabetic characters—has not, but developing a feminist theory of letters alongside embryonic material and language hints, at least, at its potential breadth of engagement.

And so, these chapters chart the slimy paths and trails of embryonic material and of script dismissed as no longer useful as well as the smeared memories that each leaves, in the form of nostalgia, in the fields and environments they have visited. They are dense, overwhelming, and hopefully absorbing—in a curiosity shop sort of way; but unless you have bought what the first two, theoretical chapters are selling, unless you have already invested in the initial two or three objects in your collection, it is unlikely that retrieving the other, more numerous, infinite, items in the series, stretching out toward an unattainable limit point, is going to have the pull and attraction that it would if you were already infected by the collector's instinct. You have to give the feminist theory a chance in order to make the history palatable.

Perhaps a more effective means of preparing a reader for—or of exploiting a reader's vulnerabilities to—the proposals that will be popping up, optimistic and occasionally carnivalesque, over the next hundred or so pages, is therefore to pause to reflect on the methodologies at play here. How does the mechanism that keeps these proposals in badly oxidized, jerking rotation not grind to a halt? Since the bit after the colon in titles of academic books is nearly always more explanatory than the catchy bit at the top of the cover, consider for a moment, then, what it means to write "a reproductive history of the nonhuman." Simply, this book is a history (and a secret politics) of something called "reproduction." The basic methodological frameworks are those culled, like badgers (but don't worry—they get moved, in pretty padded trucks, to a much nicer habitat afterward), from these classic fields. Historians have dealt with reproduction; political theorists have dealt with reproduction; this book is part of that grand tradition.

In general, therefore, the first two, shorter, chapters of the book draw on political theory, while the second two, longer, chapters draw on history. The first chapter, moreover, is an extended dialogue with feminist political theory—an attempt to describe to the reader how feminist theorists have understood the posthuman and the politics of life, and what the stakes have been in such conversations. The method, generally, is to present a major question motivating feminist conversations about nonhuman biopolitics, to explore pre-existing responses to this question, and then to describe, generally, how these approaches to the question can help readers to understand the nostalgic force of this politics. The second chapter, in turn, is an extended definition of nostalgia, couched this time in more mainstream political and literary theory. It does a bit of violence to the scholarship on nostalgia—none of which considers or even begins to wonder about any nonhuman or posthuman politics of the illness, experience, state, or literary device. But in the process, this chapter also demonstrates that the methods developed by feminist theorists to address related problems in biopolitics and posthuman studies are more than capable of addressing problems like nostalgia—that, in fact, nonhuman nostalgia might be best approached as a feminist issue.

In short then, fair warning. Readers might experience some methodological vertigo as they move from the first two, relatively spare and clean, theoretical chapters to the shaggy, overstuffed case study chapters that follow. These second two chapters—taking embryos and alphabets as useful and entertaining examples—after all, draw on classic, old-fashioned historical methods not known for their excising of irrelevant, but interesting, detail (I've cited Ernst Kantorowicz in here somewhere, just to make the footnoted point). These chapters, to put it differently, are deductive—in the best and also in the most wearisome sense of the term. The result of scuttling around in archives, collecting self-indulgently massive piles of pages, passages, bits of words, words, words from documents, manuscripts, and quite nicely printed books that were, however, justifiably put to rest a century or more ago, these chapters are physically—if, by some bizarre, temporal fluke, you are actually reading a printed copy of this book—heavy.

Theorists of varied stripes find such historical methods ugly, or at best bewildering. What's the point? The implicit claim underlying this excessive collection of text, example, exegesis, and citation, however, is that—in addition to the joy of the footnote and the pleasure of the non-discovery, of the sentence in the forgotten, completely uninfluential text, that, zombie (or vampire)-like, can now be resurrected as something important—this style of historical analysis is particularly appropriate to a study of nostalgia. It is particularly relevant to a scholarly exercise that seeks to describe a mode of existence that is, in any case, always wrapped up in piles of objects and things and words that have become influential only because they have been sitting around in a drawer, or stuffed between the pages of a book (as words do tend to be), for some indeterminate, but magically transformative, length of time. It would be misunderstanding nostalgia not to gesture, at least briefly, at the historical methods that seem most congenial to it. When you bring them out into the cold, clear light of the political theorist's laboratory, as everyone knows, they just crumble into dust, or flitter out the window on bat-like wings when everyone else is looking in the other direction.

For what it's worth, historians themselves will likely also have a methodological axe to grind, or at least an axe to swing around and get caught up in the rusty gears of the rotating mechanism, as they read through these pages. How, they will ask, could a book so intent on collecting in one place this fascinating collection of citations fail, at the same time, so utterly to contextualize this collection in some coherent, perhaps nation-state specific, framework? The author could at least provide an explicit periodization. This contextualization and periodization will happen once, now, and will not happen again over the remainder of this study; so if you like that sort of thing, pay attention: most of the first case study chapter (on embryos) draws on literature in French written between the mid-eighteenth and mid-twentieth centuries (with a few outliers from other times and places as well); most of the second case study chapter (on alphabets) draws on literature in Ottoman and modern Turkish written between the mid-nineteenth and mid-twentieth centuries (with, again, the same few outliers).

Call this book, therefore, if you would like, a study of modern European history—and take methodological pleasure in the fact that this modern European history is situated in one example from the so-called center of the region, and one example from the so-called periphery. Go read some Pheng Cheah to figure out which example is which.[47] Once again, the context and period are not the point of the study—but if anyone wants to have a fight about that, a case for the choice of literature, the relevance of its national, cultural, geopolitical, and temporal provenance, can easily be made. There was a raging industry for that in the late 1990s.[48] But far more useful, to understand the spirit of the book, is to appreciate each, decontextualized object or bit of information, absent era, for its own sake, for its *failure* to relate to any coherent, well-collated whole.

Finally, an even better place to end this manipulative plea to keep reading (just skip the pages that are omitted from the preview—it won't make a difference) is with a note on style. This book is overwritten. In fact, I'm going to draw away the curtain (already in tatters) separating reader from author and tell you, the reader, that when I, the author, sent passages of this manuscript to colleagues (the gentler ones) for comment, they not so gently asked me whether I had developed a professional death wish in presenting my research like this. A death drive, maybe (read the book). But here is the problem: there is something sad as well as disingenuous about presenting an argument to a reader—about presenting a work of feminist theory to a reader—on reproduction, repetition, growth, flourishing, thought, life, memory, affect, sensitivity, and nostalgia in the short, telegraphic sentences that make for good clear analysis.

The only way to do justice to both the topic of the book and the methodological initiative it undertakes is to let go and take pleasure in an impressionistic and associative play of words. Rosi Braidotti put it much better, a number of years ago: "My hope is that what appears to be lost in terms of coherence can be compensated for by inspirational force and an energizing pull away from binary schemes, judgemental postures, and the temptation of nostalgia."[49] Much of the rest of the book deals with temptation and nostalgia—hold off on comment for now. The idea that resonates here is that stylistic "coherence" is a bad fit—in the language of that other, unmentionable sphere of academia-as-profession—for certain genres of humanistic study; this book falls into one of those genres.

So take my word for it, the fact that the writing and argument meander and bend back on one another, the fact that linear logic is not a prominent rhetorical device in these pages, does not mean that the study lacks rigor. Every bit of erratic punctuation—every dash, every colon (even the parentheticals)—every mixed metaphor galloping off of the page, every extended, tenuous sentence, complete with dangerously dangling, hanging clauses and participles, has been carefully, vigilantly composed. That sentence just took 50 minutes to write. If the prose seems lazy or easy, that's perfectly fine: let it flow over you and enjoy it. If, contrarily, it seems painful and tortured, that's good as well. These assemblages and accumulations of matter and data grow in such tortured ways—"vibrant," maybe, but certainly not carefree. Have you looked recently at a weed struggling up through the soil in your bed of kale and nasturtiums, only to be ripped out at the first moment it feels the sun, at the mold on your stale bread shrinking away from the accidental splash from your environmentally friendly kitchen soap, at the code that went into the graphics representing your online shopping cart, now crashed? They are no more spare and elegant than the sliced up, vanishing embryos in the Blechschmidt collection. But still, nonetheless, you should at least spend a moment to look at them.

Feminist Theory and
the Politics of Life

Pretend that in the far corner of the model room, next to one of the less well known and well regarded sculpted embryos, an unobtrusive music ensemble is playing. Something mathematical—Bach or bluegrass. The occasion is unimportant—let's say they were hired to celebrate the triumphant return of the collection from its incarceration at the Carnegie, to serenade the specimens home. Having established motivation, the crucial concern here is that the music is contrapuntal, winding its way through a backdrop and foreground of embryos and embryonic material extending toward a vanishing point. That is the sensory climate hovering over the current chapter. The embryos remain. But plinking and tapping against their glass and plastic enclosures are the notes of a musical conversation between two fields whose convergence can be both disconcerting and, if done right, chillingly (or, depending on your politics, tinglingly) effective.

Here, the exchange is between variations on feminist theory and variations on biology and neurophysiology. Elizabeth Grosz is reading Darwin alongside Rudolf Leuckart, Claire Colebrook is in conversation with *Cell*, and Rosi Braidotti is writing of consciousness alongside Alain Prochiantz writing likewise on cerebral plasticity. The purpose of this, however, is not to make some claim about feminist clarifications of, or challenges to, neuroscience. The scientists are safe. Rather, as bits and pieces of— or deliberate detritus from—the past hundred fifty years of biology come into contact with the past two to three decades of feminist political theory, a useful mirror image of Foucault's biopolitics inches, blurry, into the frame. The feminist theory and the often speculative biology integrate into a nonhuman biopolitics in which reproduction gives way to thought. Still, despite the music, don't lose site of the embryos.

Foucault himself never did. Creeping out of the cracks and crevices of his politics of life—this politics, ordinarily, of bounded bodies, embodied subjects, and disciplined selves whose health, sexuality, and reproduction translated inexorably into bound and massive nation-states, flourishing bodies politic, and obese popular governance (birthing in the process a late twentieth-century glut or gluttony of scholarship on thanatobiopolitics, out to reveal the horror of a flourishing life that eventually rots)—have always been morsels and fragments of unbounded, disembodied, radically undisciplined bits, bytes, and flickers of systems. As the classic biopolitical humans—embodied, disciplined, regulated, and reproducing—performed their quotidian biopolitical task, other elements of Foucault's life- and environment-obsessed politics of democracy and vitality outstripped their humanesque models.

Consider, for example, the statistical apparatuses, replicating, copying, and achieving an emphatically non-metaphorical life of their own, producing a quite literal plethora of data. Statistics are central to Foucauldian biopolitical theory,[1] but play in post-Foucauldian scholarship, despite their remarkable reproductive capacity, sexual second fiddle to the human body rarely at rest.[2] Or consider the environment—that modern biopolitical fixation on organic systems as well as the insidious toxicity that weakens them, or that leaves them lethargic, luring them away from their life-sustaining role. It is difficult to shunt and crush these systems of information and matter and into the human-fixated conventional theories of political life (or political life as, not so secretly, death) that have claimed to take Foucault as a starting point. But there is no reason why one ought to. Yes, Foucault liked his human bodies. But his theory of biopolitics is, already, as written, in its finite form, also replete with *non*human nonbodies reflecting both life and the politics of life.

Nonetheless, as Hannah Landecker has noted, Foucault drew on nineteenth century, not twentieth century, not to mention twenty-first century, life sciences as he fleshed out his tale of biopolitical life and reproduction.[3] His work is not known for its cutting edge references to molecular biology. Or, as Rosi Braidotti put it ten years before Landecker floated her gentler critique, whereas someone like Donna Haraway can ground her claims concerning the politics of life—and its odd, relentlessly nonhuman symptomology—in a formal study of biology, Foucault was no scientist (not to mention being "intrinsically androcentric").[4] There is thus something lacking in Foucauldian biopolitics—and this is undoubtedly also the something that opened up that tempting empty maw into which the death-obsessed theorists of 1990s "life" repeatedly cannonballed. There is an artificiality, a bit of accidental plastic plant life, acting as a frustrating barrier in Foucauldian biopolitics among the life of accumulating information, the life of unbounded organic systems, and the life of that battered, bounded human body.

This is not, though, once again, because nonhuman assemblages weren't integrated into Foucault's original articulation of biopolitical democracy. There is ample evidence throughout his work that lush data as well as environments run rampant were as central to his politics of life as human selves and subjects were.[5] Foucauldian biopolitics has always been at least in part nonhuman. What it has not been, however, is nostalgic. Or, to start with the more general point, this point that pierces its way through this and later chapters: an issue that does fail to feature in Foucault's writing, and an issue that has blossomed and flourished in the sciences since Foucault wrote (although, once more, it was there, dormant, long before his time), is the intellectual life lived by organic material and informational systems. This intellectual life—of unbounded accumulations, systems, growths, and fields of matter and data—has fruitfully seduced recent biological writing, to the extent that this writing has on occasion resuscitated, even if inadvertently, oddly anachronistic themes floated by long-dead, eighteenth- and nineteenth-century cranks (or were they?) on the thought of assemblages, and on reproduction as contemplation.

Cellular decision-making, choice, and sensitivity in fact dart about in increasing profusion nowadays across wildly varied scientific fields, alongside models of life that replace boring, bounded bodies with accumulations, growths, assemblages, and environments.[6] Living, in recent biological work, has both expanded beyond bodily boundaries and become, itself, thinking. Rather than arbitrarily assigning certain bodies the spotlight role of thinking organic whole and certain other, more abject bodies the role of unthinking, affectless part, many of these papers treat life as a series of interconnected systems, collectively deciding, thinking, feeling, or meditating.[7] "Life," so defined, is a set of infinitely divisible parts that think as they process, interact, integrate, and disintegrate.

Notice the absence of cognition here—embodied, fractured, distributed, extended, or otherwise. But fear not: its exclusion from this brief, evocative, but not even close to exhaustive rehearsal of a tidal wave trend in neurophysiology and life science is not a mental tic, an irrational or neurotic bit of symptomatic forgetfulness. On the contrary, cognition in this research—as well as in the squelched early-nineteenth-century writing that it eerily echoes—is very much an afterthought. No Prometheus or Procrustes in sight. Indeed, the thought that overlays life in this work is an activity, not a formulation. It operates, hums along to itself, rather than throwing up, vomiting up, glorious abstract absolutes. It decides, chooses, senses, remembers, feels, and intuits. No cognition, no brain, no consciousness of self, no consciousness of other, no hyperactive theory of mind stultifies the life as thought that accumulates in small hillocks in the clefts and out of the way places of these fields, systems, and environments.

Once again, however, this—intellectual—aspect of unbounded life is absent from much of Foucault's work. And it was not present, or at least not as present, in the natural sciences when Foucault wrote; the more

eccentric figures of eighteenth- and nineteenth-century biology and neuroscience were not yet sneaking out of the superfluous corners to which
they had been confined. Although data and information did live lives of
their own in Foucault's biopolitical governance, these lives did not in turn
think on their own. They were tied up with, and muffled by, the biological life and sexually reproducing bodies that generated them. In the mid-
twentieth century, when Foucault wrote, natural scientists concerned with
life and reproduction were not, for the most part, equally concerned with
thought—and neither was he.

But this doesn't mean that Foucault's biopolitical theory is now an
artifact, a relic, something to wrap up in plastic and place among the
Blechschmidt models. If anything, the recent scientific work on nonhuman thought as nonhuman life, makes explicit the implicit yet evocative
and haunting connections in Foucault's theorization between, on the one
hand, information, processing, and environments, and on the other hand,
biological life, reproduction, and embodied matter. There is nothing in
recent scientific research that undermines Foucauldian theories of biopolitical mass democracy. On the contrary, this research harmonizes with
it. Or, as feminist theorists of nonhuman biopolitics have already hinted,
the politics of life, formulated by Foucault or otherwise, can easily stretch
from bodies to material assemblages to fields of data, endlessly processing.

So what comes now is the contrapuntal exchange—the cord (chord)
that winds its way through the embryonic display. Its austere and minimal
starting point is an obscure nineteenth-century laboratory, madly creating
life, life, life—life as thought—which will give way, inexorably, to a series
of feminist theorists who have found fermenting in these and other petri
dishes the moldy building blocks of a nonhuman biopolitics. Its final set
of variations and deviations will be a set of similar interactions over the
twentieth and twenty-first centuries, followed, for kicks, with some recent
ethical dilemmas—parasites and parthenogenesis—that these deviations
have exhumed. The historical and contemporary neuroscience and the
feminist political theory are necessarily entangled.

But keep in mind as this counterpoint unfolds: this coiled loop (yes,
the metaphor has teetered and now completely shifted from music to

weaving—but think Circe if it makes you feel better, since we are heading back to nostalgia eventually)[8] of science, science studies, feminist theory, and political theory, unravelling and stitched back together again (now think Penelope), serves a single purpose. It eventually forms a net—if a frayed and disintegrating one—in which to hold a theory of nonhuman biopolitics that can become a theory of nonhuman biopolitical nostalgia. The chapter is dishonest. Even as it demonstrates the validity of a politics of life identical to a politics of thought, even as it carefully constructs an argument in support of biopolitical reproduction as biopolitical contemplation, its gaze is fixed elsewhere, in deliberate misdirection. And the rabbit is actually a conclusion concerning the affective nostalgic quality of nonhuman organic and inorganic political participation—via replication, via reproduction, via growth.

Perfect departure point: parts and wholes prior to Darwin's 1859 defeat of Platonic perfection. Reading Rudolf Leuckart's 1851 *Polymorphismus der Individuen*, Lynn K. Nyhart and Scott Lidgard find an early-nineteenth-century natural historian concerned with how to define the organic, living "individual," and thus how to recognize threats to unitary life in biology.[9] Leuckart, they write, mourned—even before Darwin dealt it its death blow—the classical definition of the individual as the worldly reflection of ideal "kind" or "type," and he (Leuckart) thus shied away from morphology or physiology as indicators of living totality or wholeness.[10] Leuckart's leap, however, from this place of melancholy was not into endless, frustrating, reactionary abstraction, but rather into a madcap, modern, and emphatically non-classical reconsideration of the relationship between organic reproduction, especially, and individualized versus undifferentiated life—between replication, growth, and flourishing, on the one hand, and defining part and whole on the other.

And how relevant were his conclusions? First, according to Nyhart and Lidgard, he chipped away at "the hegemony of sexual reproduction"—linked inevitably to bodily individualization—by invoking, along, it is true, with many of his contemporaries, the more empirically verifiable dominion (more forceful than hegemony) of other types of replication, of "alternation of generations, parthenogenesis, and hermaphroditic reproduction."[11] From that murky place of churning, inseparable creation, absent any hint of part *or* of whole, Leuckart took another step away from life initiated in the discrete body and toward life as an accumulation of roiling matter. He equated reproduction, in any form, with a panoply of other material needs or desires, from moving to eating to sensing to defecating.[12] All reproduction, all generation, all initiation of vitality pirouetted on a continuum with all facets of the maintenance of life, the initiation of life "neither mysterious nor special."[13] Sexual reproduction, an initiating act, associated always with unitary, embodied wholes—and diverging always, in this singularity, from every other living activity, especially thinking or meditating—stepped to the side in favor of flourishing, fecund, generation as growth.

In response to the (political) trauma that was the death of the classical abstract, ideal type with its imperfect material echo or embodiment—not to mention the attendant birth and growth of fuzzy matter and information around formerly clear cut, and cut clear, now dead, parts and wholes—Leuckart redefined biological life and reproduction. The antidote to his political longing was a total immersion in the muck of an alternative biology. In place of individual bodies reproducing (imperfect) echoes or models of perfect types, Leuckart imagined nonhuman, not even close to human, accumulations that generated as they moved, consumed, excreted, and felt. There is a budding biopolitics here of unbounded, disembodied organic matter—a politics of reproduction that is also everything else in life. But is it a biopolitics of thought? Implicitly, of course, if reproduction is everything that living matter does, then it is also thought. But this association does not become explicit in Nyhart's and Lidgard's reading of Leuckart.

It does, though, become explicit in Elizabeth Grosz's treatment of Charles Darwin alongside Henri Bergson and Gilles Deleuze.[14] Grosz's sympathetic take on Darwin's theories of life leaves a scholar sheepish about fitting out (as I just did in my reading of Nyhart and Lidgard on Leuckart) this superstar of natural historians, the biologist who changed everything, as the intellectual executioner of his misguided, if well intentioned, predecessors.[15] Grosz, for example, compellingly downplays the faintly disreputable (at least in some quarters[16]) gratification Darwin felt toward discrete, if complex, bodies—backward echo of Foucault—and the linear (sexual) inheritance of traits that go with them.

Yes, Grosz writes, Darwin trades on enclosed wholes with distinguishable outsides and insides; his books are brimming with borders and membranes.[17] But, far more important to his general theory of life—and in harmony with the less completion-obsessed Deleuze and Bergson—are, first, his insistence that what "makes a living being a cohesive whole" are "the peristaltic forces of cohesion and disintegration," and second, his proposition that life writ large is a "contained dynamism," "porous," a "complex fold of the chemical and physical that reveals something not given within them, something new, an emergence, the ordered force of invention."[18] Important to Darwin, in other words, as much as it had been for Leuckart, was a living norm that was boundless, generative, and generating—a sort of endless slime. Less key was a life that was singularly reproductive, or the product—like humans—of acts that easily discriminate between and among wholes (in turn composed of parts). Life, for Darwin, according to Grosz, was characterized by dynamism and sets of relations rather than by static bodies arrayed in an endless, un-frayed line of undeviating inheritance.

Downplaying Darwin's delight in whole, sexually reproductive organisms in this way, Grosz domesticates him—demonstrating his affinity both to less celebrated earlier natural historians like Leuckart and to infinitely more respectable (again, at least in some quarters) figures like Deleuze. Grosz follows a fascinating thread, a thin filament from Darwin as a proponent of dissolved membranes and non-sexually reproductive matter-as-Life to Deleuze describing a life that exceeds particularity, that is "lived in excess of a subject, beyond consciousness," "a singularity without identity," and that thus shares "living" not just with other matter and information but with "nonliving events," "unpredictable emergences," "the weather, the ocean, gravitational forces," and "nonliving forces" generally.[19]

Darwin the celebrity in this way does take something of a beating in Grosz's book—he is anything but the unique creative genius whose brilliant thought changed the world. But Darwin the theorist of life with the shocking—no, no that wasn't supposed to happen, stupid, stupid Herbert Spencer[20]—political afterimage also becomes infinitely more palatable. Rather than mad, bad demographic engineers abusing poor Darwin's science in order to produce a century and a half of mass death, Darwin's discoveries instead, via Grosz's reading, become the playthings of an *alternative* political theory. He can relax, albeit awkwardly, and undoubtedly with some confusion, among the Victorian thinkers who perhaps weren't immediately responsible for the horrors of the twentieth century. As one of many nineteenth-century biologists who defined life as dynamism, as a series of unpredictable, generative relations and interactions, Darwin in this re-telling of the story helps to initiate a politics of boundless life—and also a politics of reproduction as thought.

Grosz continues, for example, still reading Bergson, Darwin, and Deleuze together, that given this substitute—yet evocative—definition of life, political thought also changes radically. The yearning to overcome difference, to unify, to identify the ideal, to distinguish parts in order to form them into satisfying wholes, to feel the gratifying release of the abstract, dissipates.[21] There is no "overcoming" of "differences" in the name "of a universal term"[22] in the politics that emerges, limping, dripping—yet at least not lashing out in resentful, racist frustration—from this theory of life. Rather, this alternative politics of boundless, nonhuman life, once it has rested on the shore a moment, engulfs and consumes and excretes out into formless lumps of information and matter even the tiniest traces of what was once abstract, unitary, unifying ideal thought. The particular overruns all here—and "difference generates further difference because difference makes inherent the force of duration (becoming and unbecoming) in all things, in all acts of differentiation, and in all things thus differentiated."[23]

So obviously Leuckart slaked his melancholy, seemingly unquenchable thirst for a classical politics of abstract thought and identifiable, individual wholes with a dip in the puddle of fecund, flourishing, non-sexual, yet radically reproductive slime. That's where his replacement politics sat, budding, opening out, preparing itself, waiting for a twentieth-century carnival of mass democracy and of mass surplus—but not, emphatically, of mass death. If Darwin's work (standing in for the work of countless frenetic philosophers of the stuff that grows on the underside of the Blechschmidt Collection's plastic containers, the part that doesn't get cleaned as often as the rest) lends itself to a politics of unbounded, nonhuman life, then, as Grosz writes, a quite specific regime of *thought* also takes command. Life becomes a variation on one very distinctive, focused mode of thinking—thought in the particular, in the concrete, in the drastically anti-abstract. Bergson, for example, "anticipat[ing]" a great deal of recent theoretical biology, described not only the "capacity for 'choice'" in even "the most elementary forms of mobile life," but he also argued that this choice, this thought, this consciousness "expresses both the particularity of each species and the specificity of individuals within them."[24] As assembled stuff, writ large, via its particularity, lives, so too does it think.

Or, more pointedly (yes, back to the perforating point—don't think that the music has stopped) Grosz, following Deleuze, argues that as much as both this flourishing life and flourishing thought take shape (or shapelessness) through repetition, repetition is not identity. Repetition does not perpetuate unity. On the contrary, one of the most glaring examples of repetition gone awry, of repetition absent identity, of the distinction between the particularity that is life and the sterility of unitary, abstract cognition is, revealingly, memory. "Memory," she writes, is not "added to each perception," but rather "each perception inheres in an order of the virtual that expands and elaborates it through its difference from, and thus in its addition to, each earlier repetition."[25]

Memory is linked to "the living," in other words, and a quite effective definition of the "nonliving," in turn, is, for Grosz, existence absent memory: "the living," unlike the nonliving, enjoy (if we're being optimistic) "the continuous growth and accumulation of the past, through their inherent immersion in virtuality."[26] More on memory, itself, in the next chapter. For now, it is sufficient to present a hypothesis: it seems that when nineteenth-century biologists serve as guides, they blaze a scorched earth trail toward a politics of life in which the defining characteristic of being alive is, specifically, enjoying a repetition (reproduction) that is not just thought, but also memory. Living, for them, is remembering (and thereby reproducing). Not living is—not.

So, thus far, historically (we'll get to a few examples from contemporary biology soon): Leuckart and his goo, along with Darwin and his many disciples, as read by Grosz, have at the very least created the conditions for a nonhuman biopolitics. They have made possible a nonhuman thought mapped onto nonhuman life and reproduction, a thought that is always embedded and anti-abstract. What, though, are the implications of a living norm that is explicitly nonhuman and of a reproduction that is identical to thought? And what are the implications of allowing memory, especially, to saturate these proto-political tales of freakishly successful variations on life?

In volumes one and two of her "Essays on Extinction,"[27] Claire Colebrook begins to untangle this nonhuman biopolitics of thought and reproduction that ties the work of nineteenth-century biologists to the writing of the twenty-first-century feminist theorists who read it. Cutting through the wooly confusion, she defines as the key characteristic of the contemporary (feminist) posthumanism that "hails an end to human exceptionalism," the dismissal of "cognition-oriented models"[28]—or, what she calls in the second volume, the "late twentieth-century anti-cognitive turn to life as vitalism."[29] The reference to the end of the last century there, just a heads up, is a way of indicating both that cognition is already in bad odor and that making a case for a politics absent this cognition, absent self-consciousness, and absent rationality—a politics that does away with discussions of identity and the Other (there's a throwback)—is already, see Žižek, out of style. That was fast. Political thought as work rather than cognition is not only well established, but open to disdain by those who've seen it and done it to death.

But Colebrook takes her discussion of nonhuman (posthuman) politics—this politics of life, death, and reproduction without bodies, corpses, or genetic legacies—on an unexpected and absorbing detour after flagging her awareness of the changes in fashion. With a brief rest stop at a question that doesn't ordinarily get a lot of attention—why hate the brain so much? (because of "a widespread anxiety regarding the brain's own capacity to destroy itself through the very perceptive power that generated its supposedly proper potentiality in the first place,"[30] leading, in turn, to meth for kids with various Cartesian deficits or surpluses[31])— Colebrook goes on to note that a useful way to re-frame the problem of posthuman politics is to address "the perception of futurity."[32] Rooted in all of the disembodied yet material vitality, all of the systemic yet non-cognitive thought, in all of the lurching variations on nonhuman bio-politics that have spurted and spouted out of this previously austere and mathematically intertwined counterpoint,[33] in other words, is a single, key strand: imagining the future. If the politics of life gets mixed up with the politics of thought (and if cognition thereby necessarily gets the chop), then proper political thought is, above all, beyond all, thought of futurity.

So Colebrook unexpectedly gives the "Cartesian 'mind'" a bit of breath-ing room. This mind can't be "nothing more than a falsehood" (a wisp of tempting certainty out to mystify those seeking out truth [or is it reality? Or fact?]) because defining it as such fails "to account for its force, its persistence, and the possible futures it presents to the organism."[34] More pointedly (yes, again), once this mind revives a bit, and takes in the air of infinite, potential, boundless futures (goals, plans, and endpoints—not the points we've been sharpening here), it lends itself to all sorts of unex-pected posthuman permutations. When, as an intuition of futurity, the Cartesian mind springs back into action—as a bit player, true—it intro-duces squarely into the biopolitical sphere, into the regime of reproduc-tion as thought, among other performers, actors, and actants, for example, the virus, which always, confusingly, straddles the fence between life and not-life. Although—missing (if not grieving) borders or membranes—the virus "cannot be defined as a form of life on the Maturana and Varela model," Colebrook can nonetheless wonder "what might the future or temporality of viral life be?"[35] With no inside or outside, no potential for "invasion" or "influx," the "virus does not have a world"—but, "in one respect," stemming from its absent relations, "it is only viral life that has a future."[36]

The politics of life, then, for Colebrook, is identical to a "politics of viral futures"; biopolitics *must* abandon "the world of the body," humans sexually reproducing themselves, in favor of boundless "life," because such life has political force only when bodies dissipate.[37] Once biopolitics does take viral life as a norm, however, it becomes a politics not just of life, but of a particular type of thought—the thought that Deleuze and Guattari defined, this thought as an "opening to the eternal," an "intuition" that "goes beyond the organism's own duration," ejecting from the life boat "'man' as isolated thinker" and making room for an apprehension of "the inorganic potentialities that exist now only in confused and all too human composites."[38] Implication number one of the historically situated biopolitical turn toward the nonhuman, the endless and boundless slime, goo, and information, then: political life inevitably gets itself all wrapped up in political thought. And political thought—Descartes and Darwin now both dusted[39] off and placed, if not on their cracked pedestals, at least at the table with the rest of us, albeit in vastly different costumes, as protoposthumanists—is an intuition of the future. Biopolitics sheds its human form quite quickly; and once the human winds up in the ditch, thought takes center stage.

Reproduction and sexuality enter the picture—stage to cinema—in this scenario as well. Colebrook invites her readers, for example, to try to "think about the sexuality of time in its capacity to create syntheses and productions beyond those of organic striving"—to appreciate the reproductive capacity of Deleuzian occasions (not just Darwinian organisms) in this detonated nonhuman biopolitics.[40] Once introduced, once shoved into the frame, this reproduction repeats (yet never identically—don't lose sight of the differences, the mutations, as the Blechschmidt embryos veer away into the vanishing point) the same haunting theme, this bit of counterpoint stuck in our collective, Cartesian, non-cognitive head (or lap).

So hum along to the nonhuman logic: this reproductive capacity eludes any "logic of sustaining or rendering ourselves viable," writes Colebrook, it refuses "life as it actually exists" in favor of "aspects of life that are not truly actualized—problems, questions, disturbances," it satisfies not via "self-recognition," but by "extending [the organism's] powers of mutation," and it replaces the energy of "living on, of sustaining, extending, [and] adapting," with a vitality "open to the forces of its own destruction."[41] Let's keep going. Rather than identifying reproduction, replication, and making copies with sustainability—albeit sustainability through instability and a healthy "alterity"—replication and reproduction are instead thoughts of the future, of time twisted backward then forward once again.[42] As Colebrook puts it, when a virus replicates itself in a body, in my body, it creates "not a different organism but a different potentiality—a new virus or the modification of an organ, which might then affect my body's motility."[43] Viral life and viral reproduction are hence politically resonant because they encounter, and think about, the future.

This is an interesting turn of events—past, present, and future tripping all over themselves when reproduction turns to thought. Grosz, for example, steps (not tripping) from nonhuman life to the nonhuman politics of life to nonhuman biopolitical thought to nonhuman biopolitical thought as memory to, finally, reproduction and replication as the crucial (yes, I'm avoiding "vital") activities in the preservation and production of this memory/thought. Colebrook does the same thing, but in place of "memory," she slips in a sense of time, "futurity." According to Grosz, reproduction is biopolitically important (vital would be really useful here) because it remembers, According to Colebrook, reproduction is biopolitically important because it senses futurity. Another quick heads up: for those not yet in the know, memory colliding with an uncanny sense of futurity is more often than not termed "nostalgia."[44]

So we might pause for a moment to appreciate the vital role that nostalgia seems, at least, to play in the historical development of biopolitics as it appears in the writing of Colebrook and Grosz. But this pause will last, truly, for just for a moment—after all, nostalgia thrives on hints, denial, and withholding; no need to divulge all (although, parenthetically, not to worry—we'll pin it down in the next chapter). All this talk of Bergson, Darwin, Descartes, Deleuze, and a bit of Nietzsche waving from the bottom, left hand corner, is fine, but it seems a bit archaic, no? Reproduction as thought—memory and a sense of futurity—is still a far cry from the conventional Foucauldian take on this fundamental biopolitical behavior when it pops up in contemporary analyses of the contemporary period, in, say, policy writing.

Yes, it is true, some have already noted the disappearance of sexuality—linear inheritance—from biopolitical governance, and its replacement by a seemingly (but hold back judgment—and don't forget Leuckart's joy in his goo) more staid focus on reproduction in and of itself, absent sex.[45] And the posthuman environment, the boundless system or network has pushed its way into, seeped across the interstices of, even the most tame and caged of biopolitical arguments. A gesture toward that rapidly receding, cringe-inducing unfashionable, vanishing posthuman moment is, right now (oops, the moment passed) de rigueur. But can we really say that contemporary biology, like its nineteenth-century counterpart—in conversation with recent feminist theory—in fact lends itself to this nonhuman biopolitics of reproduction as thought, memory, and, slyly insinuatingly, nostalgia?

Asking the question obviously presupposes the answer. Start, therefore—nodding to Leuckart—with a few scattered bits of grit from more recent scientific studies on parts, wholes, life, reproduction, thought, sensitivity. Shuffle forward, then, to the feminist writers who have—formulated is the wrong word—conjured up theories of democracy and life out of such dust motes and whirlwinds of speculative (and also, in addition, quite grounded, in the dust) biological research. From there, the running relevance of biopolitics as necessarily nonhuman, and of reproductive life as thought, as memory, comes, once more, bursting through. In a 2011 article in *Cell*, for example, Gabor Balazsi, as first author, like Colebrook, explores the odd congruence of viral reproduction and viral thought replicating, parasitizing, killing, embedded in simultaneously reproducing, replicating, living, dying, thinking organic matter. Balazsi et al. start with a set of nice, coherent, taxonomically satisfying comparisons and contrasts between bacterial and viral life, reproduction, and choice. After that, though, things start feeling a bit more post-apocalyptic.

Bacteria, for example, are offensively successful life forms—remember all of that paradigm shifting work from the early 2000s about people living in the age of bacteria, bacteria surviving without light, heat, or food that any normal organism would call "food"?[46] Head back there—Balazsi et al. tackle the question, in part, of why bacteria keep putting the rest of us to shame. In part, they write, bacteria are successful because many assign separate and distinct functions to different cellular groups within their populations, thus not only responding to, but merging with, their environments. They deal with the inherent, yet radical contradiction of being alive as both discrete individual and amorphous group not with a wild spiral into neurosis, but by enjoying their incoherence—decoherence—by exploding the whole altogether, and thus deflating completely the problem of interior and exterior. Cyanobacteria, for example, handle mutually exclusive functions—"photosynthesis and nitrogen fixation"—by assigning one part ("population") of their cells to the poisonous undertakings, while "the rest of the cells remain photosynthetic."[47] Other bacteria disintegrate along more relevant, for our purposes, cracks and fissures—separating "somatic cells" from "germ cells," and allocating "the tasks of locomotion and replication" to all sorts of varied "subpopulations."[48]

Parts and wholes, then, à la Leuckart, are something of a non-starter here. As is any attempt to pin down the bacterial individual—which, in any case, would simply ooze around, or perhaps eat, the pin—as a thinking versus replicating versus growing being (three binary sides there, but bacteria can do that). Each bacterial cell is an individual, in the possessing a membrane, making a decision to perform one function over another, sense of the term. But the bacterial population as a whole, constantly slipping into parts, constantly becoming backdrop, framework, set as well as actor and actant, makes a mockery of separating out certain—intellectual—activities from other—reproductive—activities, of trying to isolate linear reproduction, the creation of new individuals, as a uniquely important activity. Or, to twist the leftover liberal value judgment in the other direction: the reproductive germ cell houses information, a message, that might certainly be communicated or passed on, but this germ cell is neither more important, nor more relevant to theories of life writ large, larger than life, than the somatic cell. It is a germ cell rather than a somatic cell purely by accident, purely because of how the goop navigates, reproduces, or becomes, itself, an environment.

Leuckart, in short, comes back, updated, with a vengeance—the last vapor of his melancholy beading up and streaming off. But watch what happens as Balazsi et al. introduce into their analysis viruses—even less prone to reassuring genre distinctions, flickering back and forth in their frustrating way across the life/not-life, not to mention matter/not-matter (secretly information), non-boundaries, like light waves out to irritate onlookers. Viruses, according to Balazsi et al. are, as Colebrook also notes, unique living (or quasi living, or, all right, to some, not-living) organisms (or quasi organisms) because they "can only multiply inside of the cells they parasitize."[49] But in every other way, "viral decisions" are the same as "bacterial, fungal, and metazoan cellular fate choices," which—Balazsi posits—means that "cellular decision making is a misnomer. In fact, 'cellular' decisions are taken by more or less autonomous replicating systems that reside inside and manipulate the behavior of carrier cells to maximize the chance of their own propagation."[50]

Pause here for a moment and re-read that last quotation. Leuckart, Grosz reading Darwin and Deleuze, and Colebrook reading Descartes and Deleuze would be delighted by the scare quotes around "cellular." Yes, "cellular." That, right there, is biopolitical thought, nonhuman reproductive memory, and homeless viral futurity in a nutshell (or, obviously, not in a nutshell—not bounded at all, no dreams). If, as Balazsi et al. write, viral thought is similar to bacterial and other cellular thought, then the membrane supposedly separating individual cell from individual cell is even less of a border than anxious theorists worry it might be. Viral decision-making is, itself, free-floating reproduction as thought. It is also, according to Balazsi et al., a lot closer to other modes of living thought than it initially appears to be. If the sticky strand attaching viral reproduction to other reproductive life holds together, in fact, then neither reproduction nor thought have anything to do with the cell's (or two cells' or so very many cells') body or bodies. Life, reproduction, and thought become undifferentiated matter. Or, better, they become not quite matter, Leuckart's goo. And politically, in response to Leuckart's loss, reproduction remains the key to political theory (with life the rusty lock), but this reproduction is divorced from identifiable bodies and subjects, and spread out over contemplating, meditating fields of slime.

Or, we might say, it is spread across a field—or a puddle—of fluid. Luce Irigaray, decades before anyone worried about reconfiguring Darwin (he was still sturdy on his pedestal, no disfiguration yet) or telling Descartes it was safe to emerge (at worst, he was concealed, respectable, behind a Rawlsian veil) had already recognized the political significance of boundless accumulations of stuff, reproducing, replicating, and thinking. In her "Mechanics of Fluids," she first pinpoints—or sticks a pin, into a point, around which the rest coagulates and flows—the impossibility of translating the infinitely iterated particularity of replicating, dynamic matter into abstract unitary, fixed, ideals (without the Leuckartian breakdown).[51] In addition, she writes that because fluid resists "the countable," because it makes a mockery of unity and dialectic, and *because* it is "already diffuse 'in itself,'" it is one of the few political frameworks (yes, framework; think glass—glass is a fluid) that can handle life, reproduction, and thought together.[52] When that shaggy, uncomfortable, flailing, embryonic nonhuman biopolitics—that politics of reproduction as thought—flounders into the deep end, in other words, it turns out to swim quite well.

Or, to get at this point, pinpoint, via a different woven strand, more than a decade ago, in her *Metamorphoses*, Rosi Braidotti, drawing on Irigaray and Deleuze, pushed the politics of life as thought into even deeper water. Braidotti reconfigures consciousness at a more fundamental level, with more airless (in the Adrienne Rich sense[53]) depth, than Colebrook did ten years later. Agreeing, preemptively, with Colebrook that Cartesian dualism is a problem, but perhaps not the one that, yelling at each other for twenty-five years, we all think it is,[54] she writes that consciousness must be approached obliquely, sideways via "flows of variations, constantly transforming within patterns of continuity."[55] Consciousness, she continues, cannot be apprehended by simply re-configuring the mind, on the one hand, and the body, on the other;[56] it must be transplanted, embedded, allowed to creep and grow across "processes, flows," and the "in-between-status."[57]

Without revealing here her posthumanist hand (although she does that later), Braidotti comes at nonhuman life as thought (and reproduction as thought process) from a zigzag—snagging diagonally across the fabric (or sheet music) we have been traversing. Rather than thinking about, or exulting in, matter—and then, from there, trying to fit a new sort of thought into the stitch or the song—Braidotti instead reconceives thought first, and therefore, after, the politics of living matter. As she writes later on in the book, this is "not a mere reversal of the dialectics into irrationality, it is a different path of becoming."[58] Biopolitics, necessarily nonhuman, grounded in, grinding into, the dust or seabed of thought, emerges dripping from the depths here, not—as in Grosz's and Colebrook's work—because someone, at some point, really needs to come to terms with the proliferating, political stuff that is flourishing matter and information, but because someone needs, still, to figure out consciousness.

This flipped, inverted approach yields productive, provocative, and, naturally, thought provoking, results. Braidotti, too, notes that the politics of life is always slipping out of the human scene, and that, as necessarily nonhuman, life and thought continually, politically, contaminate one another. Moreover, the thought that Braidotti retrieves, dripping, from its fluid dynamism, is a thought that operates via reproduction and replication—via the "surprisingly generative" posthuman body, romping about in the "generative disorder" of "contemporary molecular biology" that, in turn, "is both echoed and implemented by the everyday 'gender trouble' going on in societies where sexed identities and organic functions are in a state of flux."[59]

More than that, though, Braidotti—with the frame still inverted and the threads and themes all snagged—is even better placed to isolate the exploded temporality that characterizes, without subjectivizing, this nonhuman biopolitical thought. Just as Grosz, later, emphasized memory, and Colebrook, even later, latched onto futurity, Braidotti asks, "what if consciousness were ultimately incapable of finding a remedy to its obscure disease, this life, this *zoe*, an impersonal force that moves us without asking for our permission to do so?"[60] She doesn't like nostalgia—more on that later—but she makes clear that the thought that goes with life, matter, and politics in flux, in dynamism, deep in the depths of Irigaray's mechanical fluid, is a thought that cannot escape the uncanny quality of time.

Or, as Jussi Parikka wrote just last year, if the line, drawn in the dust, between human and nonhuman, between organic and inorganic, gets blown, or washed, or gently lifted, away, then the puny human temporal order immediately explodes out into other times, into, in particular, in particularity, geological and technological temporality. Already, Parikka writes, in some accounts, "feminist ontology" has connected itself to "Charles Darwin's temporal ontology of open-ended becoming."[61] No surprise, then, of course, that the shape of our sheet, our field, our argument, our fabric, and our musical score is now a circle: here we are back at Darwin, revisited. Faced with feminist theory, the science (and politics) of life cracks, dissipates, and gives way to a politics of thought. But this thought has a complicated relationship with time. Time and thought (reproductive thought) are tightly bound, chained in both their Cartesian and their contemplative manifestations. But they are also constantly fighting each other—rolling around, awkwardly, on the dusty, muddy, moldy ground or in the dark, watery, gloom—and never achieving anything except, of course, nostalgia: the suppurating black eye that breaks out whenever time encounters embedded, material thought.

There are a lot of ethical repercussions that reverberate—percussive—out of this collision, out of life as thought, reproduction as a thought process, and biopolitics as a nonhuman variation on both. They'll get their turn to clash and bang in the later chapters of the book. To get at one, initial, weak or faint tapping of a single set of sticks, though—keeping time underneath the counterpoint of the biology and feminist theory that thread as both music and well composed stitches or woven strands, binding and linking up the repeating themes (and embryos!) that, in turn, are always fading out—one might face a human-centered problem that presents itself to those who take life just a little bit too seriously, and politically. Having witnessed, in other words an impressionistic set of historical collisions between biology and feminist theory—collisions that leave, in the midst of the startled, floating plaster and dust, a hint of a history of reproduction as thought—and having likewise observed contemporary permutations on the same sandy theme (a politics therefore of reproduction as thought), let's address one—offhand (this isn't the primary point of her essay)—ethical criticism of life as a parasite, a virus, the only life with a future.

And, nostalgically (because nostalgia, these days, is nothing if not lightning fast[62]), let's get at this problem by revisiting the hoary allusion that started this chapter: parts and wholes. Landecker, leaving aside the gentle critique of Foucault, launches a sharper censure of the contemporary biotech practice of "growing living cells of complex organisms outside of the body, often referred to as the *in vitro* culture of cells. Cells in this form," she states, "are maintained continuously as indefinitely self-reproducing populations (called cell lines)."[63] These cells lines, biologicals, make a Leuckartian mockery of the line between part and whole, wandering "plastic, temporally adjustable, highly autonomous," across the modern glass dishes scattered across today's lab benches, even as, Landecker continues, they pay a strangely abject homage to "the *idea* of the cell . . . with all of its fundamental-unit-of-life gravity."[64]

Oddly (or, secretly, not—given where we're taking this cell line of argument), one of the most prominent, prototypical functions of the disconnected pre-fabricated accumulation of biologicals has been to conjure up prenatal narratives, that is, narratives of vanishing embryos. "The genetic diagnosis at the core of amniocentesis," Landecker reminds her nostalgic readers, "depends on the ability to culture cells taken from the body, i.e. to grow and reproduce them *in vitro* for a certain period of time"—a reconfiguration of generating, growing life that rips "reproduction," as a narrative concept, almost completely out of reproductive or reproducing bodies.[65] As a result of this and other uses of disconnected cell lines, "how we handle nematode matter or yeast matter or chicken matter"—worms, mold, and birds—"may be more formative for what we do with and how we think about human matter than any particularity of human matter as human."[66]

Running relentlessly, the tapping sticks then get a bit quicker, clicking from human embryonic stuff to microscopic worms and fungus, to bits of modified bird stuff, after which Landecker finally comes to the not quite living stuff that may be the only proper model of political life. She concludes, pointedly, that experimentation on these mass produced

biologicals has made infection or "transfection" the organic norm.
"Transfection," moreover,

> is a key experimental tool for understanding how cells work, but
> increasingly the emphasis has been on its role in making cells do
> things they wouldn't otherwise do. In other words, parasites also see
> cells as something to transfect into, [and] there is a certain adoption
> of the parasite's point of view in regarding cells and the plants or
> animals they constitute as DNA and protein factories.[67]

Obliterating the distinction between parts and wholes, in other words,
leaves fuzzy at best, first, any bodily, bounded variation on reproduction
and, second, any clear borders among human, yeast, worm, and chicken
(the chicken clearly the most chilling). Most troubling, though, these new
definitions of life, reproduction, and thought force observers to adopt "the
parasite's" or the "virus's" point of view, generally, on life.

One doesn't ordinarily associate viruses with the visual scrutiny or
supervision of grand issues like existence and reproduction—with the
surveilling survival. But let's go with this proposal that the viral gaze, parasitic, is the gaze of the future. Landecker's reaction to this eventuality
is, it is true, critical (although certainly not condemnatory). A number
of theorists, though, in addition to Colebrook and Braidotti, have toyed
with taking the multitudinous, fractal eyes of the viral gaze (if we imagine
them looking, surely it can't be with two, tired lenses)—with viral life and
thought—as a less gloomy, even cheerful, norm. Myra J. Hird, for example,
has written that "engaging seriously with ... bacteria," and "theoriz[ing]
an ethics—outside pathogen histories and characterizations—that engages
seriously with the microcosms," is a worthwhile endeavor.[68] Look at them
under a microscope (keeping in mind that they may be looking back at
you)—they really are engaging organisms. The ethical repercussions of the
historical and political themes that have wound throughout this chapter
are, in other words, ambiguous at best.

One potential benefit of embracing, without hesitation, the ethical value of the viral viewpoint, for example, is that it spins out Grosz's

re-fabricated Darwin in even greater detail and texture. There is no neo-(or is it non?) Darwinian privileging of genetic information over matter or material environments[69] in this parasitic political milieu. On the contrary, viral information (or for that matter [that was deliberate] germ-plasm) is detached (unlike Darwin—nostalgia can only do so much) from its questionable colonial connotations and recuperated as a mild, if flourishing, living environment. Viral operations are not *just* the creepy alien aggression beloved of speculative fiction, the imperial infection that aids (genetic) information transmission; they are also constructive—and contemplative. They build living, thinking, reproducing, remembering fields, accumulations, and assemblages. And, as a result (of taking the viral viewpoint as a norm; not embracing infection ourselves, our bodies), the tradition that privileges the "communication" part of viral behavior over the "matter" or "thought" part of viral behavior unravels, dissipates, and disperses into dust.

But this dissipation and dust depend on adopting the parasite's point of view—on re-considering, gently, that relentless string of code out to replicate at all costs, out to force cells and self-contained bodies to do things they would not ordinarily do (out, bluntly, and without a point, to impose its domineering Cartesian thought on abject Cartesian matter). It only swirls into being if Hird (as current example) is correct: there are hidden, microscopic benefits to adopting the parasite's point of view—not least of which is recognizing life as thought and reproduction as a thought operation. Luciana Parisi has staked out the ethical work that must be done—across the whirling dust motes, musical notes, and bits of fabric—upon this adoption quite effectively: "the evolutionary model of sexual reproduction . . . needs to be re-worked through the far-from-equilibrium dynamics of molecular selection and the symbiotic networks of cellular bodies."[70]

Reproductive life needs to be defined less as an always frustrating, futile, misfired process of preserving "individual variations through sexual reproduction (genetic inheritance)," and more as a type of thoughtful action, distributed throughout an organic or inorganic environment—the "cloning of bacterial variations enfolded in every cellular and multi-cellular body."[71] The inevitable nostalgia of amniocentesis rests, then, less in the future body that those madly proliferating cells, disconnected, diverted, walled off forever, will never create than it does in the thoughtful growth of the biologicals themselves, in the reproductive contemplation, always absent any goal.

And, yet another return, this thought about the ethics—not to mention the history and politics—of biologicals would be a salve to Leuckart's psychic wounds. Nineteenth-century theories of life and reproduction—the pre-1859 and post-1859 *Origin* line now a smudged up, disfigured lack of a line in sand or water, fluid or dust—taken up and re-read by late-twentieth- and twenty-first-century feminist theorists depicts, picked out in woven strands, a deep political history not just of life, but of a non-human concurrence of life, reproduction, and thought. Contemporary biological work—exemplified, true, by a few bits and pieces of shining brushwork, integrated into the whole—likewise read by feminist theorists paints an extensive politics of nonhuman life, reproduction, and thought—with similarly extensive ethical implications. Biopolitics is, in the still floating particles of this collision, potentially and inevitably a nonhuman affair. Replicating life, reproduction, is equally inevitably thought that is a twisted, warped, tortured, but somehow still satisfying, thought about time. Memory, futurity, the geological dust of *ages* all leaving their trace residue across these various statements on thinking matter.

If there's a contribution to be made here, then, it is to demonstrate that this thought—this reproductive activity, this life, generating and flourishing—is not just memory, not just a sense of futurity, not just a sense of the agelessness of time, but the sickly, sticky state that is nostalgia. The music ensemble, exhausted, has packed up the instruments and left. The fabric—musical or woven—is a tangled mess, open neither to Circe's raveling nor Penelope's unravelling. It is snarled beyond recognition. But the embryos in the collection remain, coldly, darkly, fading into the recesses of the elongated model room. Nostalgia is a cozy state of being, at least for sliced up embryos. But it is also elusive and chilly. There is no linearity to nostalgia, as its time that never happened shrieks into the void of its time that never will be. Embodied subjects, indeed—as many political theorists have already noted—might want to reconsider the price they pay for the undoubted pleasure of nostalgic recognition. Reproducing assemblages, however, sliced ever thinner and replicating beyond recognition into geological, digital, technological time, need not necessarily concern themselves. On the contrary, they seem capable of achieving a certain suspicious synchronicity with nostalgia—as, themselves, biopolitical subjects. Or, at least, that is the thesis of the following chapter.

Nonhuman Nostalgia

Music is particularly guilty—almost worse than scent (a faultless accident of amygdalar placement)—of whistling up the eerie affect and absent, intangible half-memory that is nostalgia. Let's continue, therefore, with the homecoming concert in the Blechschmidt collection. This time, though, rather than chasing the actual contrapuntal themes that accumulated around the sliced up, vanishing embryos, listen for their echo, faint and reverberating, pinging back and forth between the dark glass or plastic, and now not quite transparent, display boxes, resting since the musicians have gone home for the night. Try—and fail—to remember the ephemeral song. It won't work—although it will leave an ache, a hollow spot. The purpose of this chapter is to probe that hollow spot. In addition to investigating the wound, however, we're also going to ask a question about it: could it be that the source of the ache is not the too human quality of the nostalgic encounter (or lack thereof), but instead the fact that nostalgia, after all, is an awkward fit for human thought, human life, and human time?

Poets, political theorists, and philosophers despise nostalgia. But this visceral—aching, perhaps—hatred may derive more from the scratchy, constricted, irritating, unbreathable (not in the Adrienne Rich sense), bad fit between human subject and nostalgic thought than from the human quality of this state. It may not be, in other words, that nostalgia, in and of itself, is at fault for the conceptual abyss into which human subjects tumble when faced with it. And so, over the following pages, let's tease out nostalgia as a nonhuman vice (or indulgence). Observe it leaking out of nonhuman life, thought, and reproduction, rather than springing up from a neurotic human need to flush out, shoot down, and then nail to a wall, lost time.

Start with a series of theorists despising the nostalgic state—not to criticize said theorists nor to point out, piously, the error of their ways, but rather to pin point (there go the pins again—pointless in the midst of memory's wisps) how nostalgia does seem to serve humans badly, with a barely concealed smirk, and thus what the defining qualities of human as well as, potentially, nonhuman nostalgia might be. From there we can traverse a few tales of nostalgia recuperated—there are more than you might think; it seems that as soon as scholars turn their startled gaze to nostalgia—as an object of study, obviously—they are transfixed, converted into apologists for this inappropriate, awkward condition, even as the sweet, sticky syrup starts to rise up around their sodden ankles. The purpose of this second stroll through the literature will be the same: What are the characteristics of nostalgia—human as well as not—in these apologetic accounts of the feeling or state as not so bad after all?

Then come three, slightly shrill (but imagine the shrillness as a distant train whistle or a tea kettle in the next, cozy, disreputably comfortable room, thereby remaining in keeping with the theme), sets of claims. First, in the abstract (or, alongside the abstract—like embedded, material consciousness, nostalgia never quite transcends the mire of the particular in favor of the purity of the ideal), nonhuman memory adheres more harmoniously than human memory does to these defining qualities of the nostalgic state, condition, position. Second, drawing once again, on a few sketchy and dissatisfying—but, one hopes, evocative and echoing—passages of a recent work of cell biology (this time around, Dennis Bray's *Wetware*), nonhuman thought and reproduction in general do lend themselves to re-definition as, narrowly, nostalgia. And finally, third—in preparation for the extended chapters on embryos and alphabets—this nonhuman reproduction as nonhuman thought that historically, politically, and ethically anchors, and has anchored, biopolitics is also, inevitably, itself, nostalgia.

Rosi Braidotti's political philosophy and style of engagement have inspired much of what is going on in this book. Braidotti, however, also is leery of nostalgia—a state she describes as both "politically conservative" and "a deterrent to serious analysis of contemporary culture."[1] Instead of contradicting Braidotti's argument—an impossibility in any case given the creepy persistence of nostalgic consumption as a panacea for late-liberal, post-liberal, did it ever even exist liberal malaise—a quick reconfiguration of nostalgia, within her own fluid framework (still glass) is a better idea. Braidotti, therefore, equates nostalgia with utopia—neither nostalgia nor utopia, she writes, "will do"[2] because, implicitly at least, neither is embedded in any sort of matter or flow.

Utopia is notoriously and etymologically (or, at least, neo-etymologically, with Thomas More in the sixteenth century writing a mere hundred or so years before the neurological invention of nostalgia, its near temporal counterpart) not a place, while nostalgia is a pain likewise detached from time. And so, rather than wrenching thought, via nostalgia, away from place and time, Braidotti writes, we should "instead linger a little longer . . . take the time to go through with these processes. Time is all one needs."[3] Might it be possible, though, to take our time while not necessarily jettisoning these timeless, placeless modes of existence (or non-existence)? Especially if we leave aside utopia (no need to disturb Prometheus or Procrustes, tired out and eviscerated from the first chapter)? Taking Braidotti at her word—agreeing, first, that nostalgia is worse than useless for humans, and second, that embedded thought and consciousness take time—might it be possible to recuperate nostalgia, to test nostalgia as a type of thought that does, after all, give us all the time in the world? This test is the trick that echoes throughout this chapter.

Simultaneously, though—time is also tricky that way—the pitfalls of nostalgic existence must also be flagged, even if these flags crack, tip over, grow moss, get buried, and wait endlessly for future archaeologists who are shocked, shocked to discover that it was New York City all the time, before they can play their cautionary role. S. D. Chrostowska, for example, in an essay on capitalism, consumption, and nostalgia plants a visible, valuable such flag, faulting the now near hysterical search for nostalgia as a type of "strip min[ing] for our past," in the name of satisfying (or never quite satisfying) a capitalist collector's instinct.[4] Yes, she writes, "depositing one's memories into the archive of culture seems the only way of preserving them from time's ravages," but as soon as these memories are transformed into collector's objects, and endowed with "excessive nostalgia," the "intimate relationship with a past" is "overwritten by abstract memories," and can lead to "gradual estrangement," obliterate any preexisting "art of decipherment," and "affor[d] us the means to ignore the radically unfamiliar and turn away from blank, unclaimed futures."[5] "At its most extreme," Chrostowska continues, nostalgia is thus "a revolt against the past as a fait accompli . . . it defies mortality and foreclosure of the possible futures it brings."[6] Finally, as a result, Chrostowska argues scholars might benefit from remembering that "modes of nostalgic experience" are "based on distinct economic models"—with the capitalist variation erupting out of "an economy of representations simulating ('retrieving,' 'repossessing') lost pasts, indeed, lost temporalities."[7]

Chrostowska's critique, then, joins, on the one hand, the mining, retrieving, possessing, collecting and archiving of specific memories, experiences, and sensitivities to, on the other hand, the destruction of personal, intimate, decipherable self-knowledge or self-care.[8] The hoard of particular memories, sense perceptions, bits of narrative that make up the nostalgic, archived collection—almost physically weighty in this analysis, straining the fingers that lug it along, and yet undecipherable in its weightiness because each bit is completely isolated from every other bit—gives way inevitably to the equally meaningless unity of the likewise

flat, abstract collection or archive as a whole. The nostalgic collection of
memories, their placement in pre-arranged, public (rather than intimate),
and therefore personally meaningless, tableaus—evoking, in a dishonest,
cheating way the thrill of the hollow ache without any actual correspond-
ing emptiness (the empty part filled, instead, perhaps with a quick squeeze
of imitation whipped cream)—is a problem because of an inappropriate
interaction between the flourishing collection of particular, dissociated
bits of stuff and the abstract narrative that fails to touch it, much less
contain it. Nostalgia—at least in its consumer capitalist connotations—is
characterized, then, metaphorically, by musical instruments, badly tuned,
giving rise to echoes that suggest, not, in fact, music, not even badly
played music, but, say, the smell of zoo animals, or someone eating an
apple; the reverberation (abstract) and the original crash (particular) are
totally unrelated.

This distillation of Chrostowska's argument resonates (that was deliberate) quite well with Jean Baudrillard's mid-twentieth-century study of
collections, nostalgia, and collections of nostalgic objects.[9] In a neurosis-
inducing assault on middle-class interior design—so much for taking pleasure in the dining table, now it's "pleasure"—Baudrillard, like
Chrostowska, ties, uncomfortably, too tightly, together the odd, indecipherable particularity of nostalgic stuff (so very many objects) with the
similarly odd, indecipherable abstractness of the nostalgic narrative (such
an endless system). Noting, for example, the synchronicity of nostalgic
furniture and nostalgic gods—a fabulous combination, lending itself to
all sorts of charming (domestic!) images of objects disporting themselves
inappropriately in posthuman living rooms—Baudrillard writes that each,
· especially, enjoys a sort of "immortality" wherein "as often with gods, furniture too . . . gets a second chance to exist, and passes from a naïve utility
into a cultural baroque."[10]

This nostalgic immortality of gods and objects, though, also gives rise to
a pernicious (or implicitly pernicious) set of deleterious effects (more on
angry gods in the ensuing chapters). After "stripp[ing]" (rather than strip-
mining, as above) "flea markets," "churches," and "museums" of nostalgic
"booty," for example, Baudrillard states that this "thirst for 'authenticity'

can now be slaked only by forgeries."[11] Even this ongoing, ultimately infinite, iteration or re-iteration of particular things and copies of things,
however, fails to satisfy the "irreversible and limitless" abstract, flattening, narrative that consumes them: "what nostalgia paints as an authentic
whole object," Baudrillard writes, "is still nothing but a combining variant
... the word 'ensemble,'" after all, "closely related to atmosphere, serves
to reintroduce any conceivable element, whatever subjective associations
it may carry, into the logic of the system ... no object can escape this
logic."[12] Even the particularity of time, broken into tinier and tinier, discrete moments, cannot, when thus objectified, evade the collector's reach.
"The watch," for example, "as an object," he finishes, "helps us to appropriate time"; and "just as the automobile 'eats up' miles, so the watch-object
eats up time. By making time into a substance that can be divided up, it
turns it into an object to be consumed."[13]

We'll revisit automotive traffic (alongside the angry gods, reclining on
their insincere furniture) in a later chapter. Here, though, to wrap up the
visceral consumption metaphors that wreck our enjoyment of the dining table we just acquired, Baudrillard, once again, comes to a compelling
conclusion. Even as countless, proliferating, distinct, particular, adamantly
physically present objects—everything from gods to furniture to forgeries
to cars to moments of time—get eaten, sucked, and inescapably drawn into
the slavering maw of the abstract, yet meaningless, system of signs, they
are never, it seems, actually digested by it. Like Chrostowska's accumulations of discrete, sensory, intimate memories that are transformed, in the
archive, in the data hoard, into nostalgic "culture," and that thereby cease
to have any relationship either to the person who ostensibly lived them or
to the narrative that issues from them[14]—infinite particularity and endless abstraction missing one another completely—so too do Baudrillard's
objects cease, even while they are being relished and consumed, to relate
to the story they tell. "Despite the thick mellow nostalgia that envelops
this 'interior,'" he writes of the restored old house, for example,

It is clear that nothing in it has the slightest symbolic value any longer.
One need only compare this description with any description of an

interior by Balzac to see that no human relationship has left its imprint on these things: everything . . . is a sign, and purely a sign. Nothing has presence, nothing has a history—even though everything is laden with references: Oriental, Scottish, early American, etc.[15]

Baudrillard's eating metaphor, then, in fact falls a little bit flat. Yes, the objects are all swallowed up, consumed, inhaled by an insatiable appetite or thirst—but after that, are they vomited up? Defecated out? Healthily digested and transformed into energy? We do know that the slavering maw itself remains unsatisfied, always hungry, suffocating, and thirsty— but Baudrillard, with his focus on the appetite loses sight of the food. Traveling, therefore, in an elementary school educational video sort of way, down into the bowels of the beast, along with the half eaten bit of matter (perhaps we can redeem the dining table after all), follow for a moment where the indecipherable goop and fluid end up once they fail so spectacularly to fill that nostalgic void.

It is true, after all, unquestionably, that nostalgic retrieval, collection, consumption, stripping, and strip mining pose a political—or political as subjective—problem. Scholars such as Chrostowska and Baudrillard are absolutely correct when they note that nostalgia divests things, objects— again, everything from sensory perceptions to a painting to a moment of time—of their subjective meaning in the name of a unitary, yet always unattainable, abstract whole. Their arguments, varied, that the trouble with nostalgia isn't just that it is sentimental, but that it traps what ought to be forward-thinking, progressive people in the past (and not even a past that necessarily occurred) are well taken. Nostalgia's pernicious, toxic quality indeed oozes just as viscous out of the gap, the failed connection, between the particular, embedded moment and the abstract, symbolic story. Poisoned in this way, people do become political subjects only with reference to flat, nonrepresentational, disengaged symbols rather than with reference to embedded objects, existence, or experiences.

But what happens to the objects (*as* objects or *as* sensory memories, experiences, embedded vitality)? They do not disappear, even as they are hoarded, reconfigured, and in fact forgotten in the name of abstract, indecipherable, disconnected narratives. Or, to get at this question (that isn't really a question) from a different, less circuitous, direction, cyano-bacteria, say, are vulnerable to different types of toxins and poisons than human subjects are. The process by which nostalgia's harrowing empty subject formation plays out—via an inappropriate, disreputable, incorrect relationship between the infinite particularity of the hoarded objects in the collection and the abstraction of the collection itself—wouldn't faze them. As terrible, psychotic, even, as this state may be for selves out to achieve (or fail, trying to achieve) psychological coherence (or an echo of such coherence), it is less of a problem for nonhumans—assemblages that might, perhaps, and justifiably, revel in the nostalgic break or fissure between particular and abstract, in the horizontal, indecipherable, iso-lated even while teeming, and never fully digested hoard or collection. The slavering, gaping maw might become, for nonhumans, perhaps, an entertaining water slide, echoing a host of vital, rather than simply senti-mental, misremembered melodies.

Intriguingly, those with a less critical attitude toward nostalgia—and even those who, despite themselves, in deliberate provocation, celebrate it—invoke the evaporating particular in the name of abstract unity (along with its deleterious psychological effects) as one of the underlying traits of this thick, mellow state. In much of this work, nostalgia *does* lend itself to zombie-like revivification (in a good way—the scholarship in this genre frequently both pro-nostalgia and pro-zombie[16])—but the infinite partic-ularity of the nostalgic state remains, obliquely, an obstacle to such recu-peration rather than the electrified fluid that makes it possible. Nostalgia may have its less toxic uses, but the gap between the abstract and the par-ticular that make the affective clock, eating time, tick is something either to avoid or to mind, specifically via reconfiguration. Embracing the gap is still, for most of these writers, not an option.

Mark Crinson's discussion of nostalgia's "uses" in mid-twentieth-century architecture, for example, historicizes beautifully the undead, monstrous, and yet oddly compelling validity of a deliberately non-critical nostal-gic take on, here, affordable housing.[17] Having bulldozed through gods, tables, paintings, cars, moments, memories, and sensory perceptions, leaving crushed bits and pieces of them scattered along the edges of the path—evocative and allusive—a swing of the wrecking ball toward buildings might be similarly edifying. Buildings, in fact, like music, are some of the nastiest culprits when it comes to lulling human subjects into a satisfying sense of (false) sentimental belonging (though mold, of course, sucks up buildings too). Crinson, however, makes a compelling case for the value, with nuance, of such saccharine structures.

Against a backdrop (modernists now themselves the flat cartoon cavorting on the dim, barely visible scrim) of modernist censure of "nostalgia," as an "escape from the present into an idealized and distorted past," as the appropriation of an "overly rosy view of the history of other people," as something "irrational," as a "distortion of history," and above all as "irrelevant to strictly architectural thinking" (in which "irony" is all right but "nostalgia," un-ironically, out of bounds), Crinson describes the, therefore, quite confrontational choice on the part of architects James Stirling and James Gowan to embrace "nostalgia" explicitly in their Lancashire housing projects (especially the Preston scheme).[18] Stirling and Gowan, Crinson continues, not only invoked nostalgia in their presentation of the Preston plan, but they did so "deliberately and very precisely," defining the "feeling" as "neither a negative concept nor a reactionary one," but rather as a means of creating "continuity with the past and offer[ing] some critical purchase on the present."[19] Or, as Patrick H. Hutton puts it in a different context, nostalgia, generally, can "disrupt continuities between past and present, redirecting human affairs in unanticipated ways"[20] (we focus here on the "unanticipated" part of his analysis, rather than on the "human affairs" part of it).

How, though, did this delicate balance between continuity and critical purchase come about? Nostalgically, first of all, by, as Crinson defines the process, "defamiliarizing devices that recalled the known but at the same time made it strange"—"reassert[ing] the past as a nonalienated relation between individual and community in the present," and thereby "restoring nostalgia's traditional links with the uncanny."[21] The sinister disconnect between particular stuff and abstract narrative—the gap between the already ugly music, haphazardly thrown together, and the echo that bears no resemblance to it—then, is key to the situatedness of a necessarily new (and, don't look, Baudrillard, soon stuffed with atmospheric ensemble pieces) plan for affordable Lancashire housing. Continuity with the past demands, in this scheme, an abstract that, yet again, refuses to talk to the particular. But this continuity, the benefits derived from the "uses of nostalgia," for the most part accrue to the buildings, to the assembled, accumulated matter and information, rather than to any actual or potential human inhabitants. The buildings—deliberately, explicitly, calculatedly haunted and new (the most chilling combination as any writer of ghost stories knows[22])—themselves delight in the uncanny. The human subjects inhabiting them may—despite going about their affairs thinking of them purely as backdrop—have a more difficult time living (coherently) with it.

In his book on nostalgia against Enlightenment (with more nuance—"nostalgia against Enlightenment" is an unfair gloss on an extraordinarily, excruciatingly [in a good way] careful study), Helmut Illbruck likewise strikes the particularity versus the abstract chord (or the particularity chord that, unresolved, gives rise to a completely unexpected, unanticipated, off key reverberation or echo in the abstract), describing nostalgia as, in part an "attachment to an incommensurable particularity of place."[23] Tracing, painstakingly, through Enlightenment era science and philosophy, interpretations of nostalgia as a disease as well as a (discredited) modern state of existence, Illbruck alights, for example, briefly on the work of Kierkegaard, noting that the nostalgic life, to Kierkegaard, like the " 'poetic' life," can be felt but not imagined.[24] Indeed, familiarly, once more, paradoxically repeating, as soon as the abstraction of poetry or nostalgia runs up against the concrete, grounded thing that is, say, "love," everything cracks, dissolves, and dissipates—"with the real interest we lose also the particular and real qualities open to temporal change."[25] Illbruck on Kierkegaard thus takes the reader even further along the pretty, detritus strewn path that beckoned at the beginning of the chapter.

Or, perhaps, try Kant. Illbruck writes that Kant's treatment of nostalgia is deep (thick and mellow, maybe), and that although he (Kant) associates nostalgia with "faulty reasoning," he also does not discount it as a state that might "have the potential to reveal something."[26] In fact, nostalgia is the product of faulty reasoning for Kant only because, narrowly, it muddles up linear temporality[27]—heaping present upon past and future, past upon present, and thus endangering the coherence of the subject. Intriguingly, though, the temporal fissures and cracks in Kant's characterization are also what make nostalgia, potentially, illuminating (avoiding, unnecessarily here, "enlightening"), especially for that purveyor of perpetual peace and limit points of future ethics and thought.[28] When nostalgia reveals (or when, to revelers in nostalgia, are revealed) impossibilities, temporal and otherwise, toward which it is proper to aspire, then the nostalgic state, reveling to the side, may actually be redeemable.

The problem—and this is important, pay attention—for Kant (and for so many others, no need to invoke Freud, he's muddling around under there in any case), therefore, crops up when, in Illbruck's words, nostalgia becomes "compulsive," or even "traumatic," when all it leads to is pointless (the points, pinging now out of the wall in a frantic heap, are back) "repetition."[29] Or, to repeat (again) it is a disease or illness, rather than a redeeming quality, especially when it calls up Baudrillard's infinitely iterated forgeries of paintings from Spanish churches cluttering up bourgeois bedrooms, or when it churns out, endlessly, Chrostowska's hoards of digital images, copied and re-copied forever in archives absent visitors. Nostalgia's poisonous erosion corrodes, then, not just when the particularity of Kierkegaard's "real" "love" (not sure where to put the scare quotes) rams up against the abstract, unifying drive of poetry and narrative, but when particularity (of any kind) sets up its own, repetitive infinity against the unitary infinity of abstract cognition—and when this repetition produces, awkwardly, a sickly kind of pleasure.

Illbruck intelligently challenges this trend in the criticism of nostalgia. In fact, he spends quite a bit of time showing that nostalgia has its value not just as a Kantian nudge in the direction of various desirable, perpetual, unattainable futures, but also in its more pernicious manifestations as compulsive repetition. Insisting that students and scholars of nostalgia remember that there has always been "a material core to it, beneath its modern intellectual history" (in its former life, especially, as an early modern neurological disease), Illbruck concludes that repetition, and most markedly, "to be repeated back into a present" might open "a future" that is worth considering.[30]

Let's go even further, though. If, as seems to be suggested by this, once again, always, impressionistic literature review, nostalgia can be defined not only by the soulless severing (if they were ever attached) of particular collected, un-collated, objects from the abstract narratives that claim to emanate from them, but also by the compulsive, sensory, and disturbingly satisfying remembering, doing, and re-experiencing of not the object and not the narrative, but rather the frayed, distressed edges of the gap between the two—if it can be defined with reference to the deep pleasure involved in repeatedly feeling the disconnect, even while swimming in the mire of matter and information—then, yes, nostalgia is not very good (despite Illbruck's well taken critique) for humans. It may be, however, the stuff of life—and of, a brief return and reminder, reproductive life, especially—for nonhuman assemblages. (Ok, and perhaps also for those rare, diseased humans not invested in their own coherent self-narrative.)

Before going in that direction, though, explore one last—in this case almost unabashedly celebratory (despite the occasional protest)—history and politics of nostalgia. In her *Future of Nostalgia*, Svetlana Boym commences her story by stating that, in its initial medical incarnation—as a "single-minded obsession" with one's "native land"[31]—nostalgia

> was not merely an expression of local longing, but a result of a new understanding of time and space that made the division into "local" and "universal" possible. The nostalgic creature has internalized this division, but instead of aspiring for the universal and the progressive he looks backward and yearns for the particular.[32]

The particular, once again, fails to speak with the abstract (universal), and thus nostalgia is born, breach. Boym, however, quickly leaves the less fruitful forest of the missed meeting between the particular and abstract in order to make her more open, field-transforming contribution to conversations, broadly, widely, about nostalgia (this contribution being to divide the state, feeling, mode of existence that is nostalgia into two types

[one positive, one negative] and then to explore the history and implications of each type).

Don't follow her into this field. It is, undoubtedly, a rich one—and certainly worth exploring—but as two and a half centuries of fairy tales have
made abundantly, lavishly clear, productive, open fields, though tempting,
lack the moody sentimental magic, the slightly acrid, sickening flourish,
of the tangled forest, the echoing contrapuntal theme. So continue exploring, but on another path that Boym reveals and begins, at least, to clear
for her readers—you can hear the faint echoes along this one. Once, for
example, she has contextualized the early modern medical diagnosis—
followed by the modern political condemnation—of nostalgia within the
false dialectic (worse than Descartes, who, despite the dusting off, would
have no idea what to do in a forest) between enlightened, modern abstract
and backward, dim particular, she presents her case for recuperating good,
"reflective" nostalgia—a style of engagement with the world that can be
"an intermediary between collective and individual recollections."[33] In the
midst of this presentation, Boym identifies a third key defining characteristic of nostalgia that will serve us well in future chapters.

Part of planting the good type of nostalgia, Boym writes, is finding the
right place to do so—indeed, given its literal (or, again, neological) meaning, nostalgia cannot be discussed *without* some critical take on place and
planting. Boym thus spends much time in her book twining up nostalgia—
good and bad—with various places, and, in particular, with various urban
places. Her field-transforming forest, in short, is a city. But the foliated
city is certainly not beyond the realm of the nostalgic fairy tale. Nostalgia
flourishes in cities with particular abandon, in fact, because of the magically, frequently paradoxical, cumulative topography of cities, because cities are often both concrete and overwhelmingly abstract,[34] because they
repeat endlessly as embedded senses, smells, and sounds even as they
assert universal coherence, and because they make a cosmopolitan claim
on the nostalgic "object of longing," which is "not really a place called
home but this sense intimacy with the world."[35] The "idea of topography,"
Boym writes, is inherently architectural in this sense—as "both a place in
discourse and a place in the world" it "is connected to the ancient Greek

art of memory," and, more so, the "mnemonic tradition recognizes the accidental and contiguous architecture of our memory and the connection between recollection and loss."[36] Nostalgic memory, encrusted all over the cities Boym visits in the book, therefore, is topographical because it celebrates the accidentally conjured up collision between an odd urban smell and its synesthetic aural echo (maybe that's the problem with the leftover music among the embryos).[37]

Or, not to mix up our senses unnecessarily, in an urban framework—the twisted arboreal foliage now nicely matted and presented under glass (still a fluid!)—nostalgia, as a *process*, rather than necessarily a state or feeling, at least as it is implicitly defined by Boym, involves spreading out or streaming stickily across a concrete (in this case, urban) environment, leaving traces of material, concrete memories of sense perceptions throughout this environment, and indeed, remembering via the debris that accumulates, repeating, but always with slight variations or mutations, across the now slimy path or gummed up system, and thereby transforming the physical place itself—here the urban network—into memory. The satisfaction and pleasure of compulsive repetition, the cloying, wan, greenish joy of re-experiencing the same, possibly completely fabricated feeling, street, bit of verbiage, or bit of foliage, does not happen simply with reference to some place or planting (that may or may not have existed in the past, present, or future); it happens via the actual, physical transformation of any place in the world, as environment, into sensory memory.

Nostalgia, then, to re-cap: is a state evanescing out of, first, the stomach churning crevice between collections of undifferentiated particularity and an abstract, unifying narrative that fails utterly to recognize this particularity; second, the ongoing, brutal, increasingly bloody and unresolved fight between the infinity that belongs to repetition or reiteration (the infinity of the particular, all nicely crammed into a tiny box, with hook and latch) and the overwhelming, soul-destroying unity of infinity in the abstract; and finally, third, the squash-plant- or slime-mold-induced transformation of physical place, system, or environment into, itself, memory—the topographical repercussions (or reverberations) of the repeated memory or experience. And finally, as a corollary, don't lose sight (smell, taste, touch, choose your mixed-up sense) of the aspect of nostalgia that leaves a bad odor, flavor, or sound in the sense organs of poets and philosophers: nostalgia also feels good. But don't be fooled: the pleasure seeping out of it is the pleasure of the uncanny, the creepy, and the haunted—of stories of things that never seem quite to die properly, of things whose vitality is, primordially, not what it should be.

Boym (as well as the others who've populated this chapter so far) insist that this nostalgia, so defined, is a solely human experience, state, feeling, or process. But whereas the others scattered across these digital pages take the humanness (or even humanity) of nostalgia as a given, Boym explicitly, and at some length, disqualifies nonhumans, and in particular machines or computers—no melancholy replicants with their dubious and thus deliciously thick (and mellow—Los Angeles does that) memories in Boym's tale—from contact with nostalgia. Depending as it does on the "materiality of place, sensual perceptions, smells, and sounds," nostalgia can survive only in a "nonvirtual low-tech world";[38] and, "like irony" (pay no attention to the fuming modernist architects in the corner), a "result of an interaction between subjects and objects, between actual landscapes and the landscapes of the mind," only "human consciousness can recognize" nostalgia, whereas computers "are notoriously lacking in affect and sense of humor."[39] The next part of this chapter will do a bit of violence to—or tag with some well-meant vandalism—this human-centered definition of nostalgic thought.

Go gently, though. In order to latch this definition of nostalgia to the nonhuman or posthuman scholarly cart, start also with a quick tour of nonhuman memory writ large, turn then to nonhuman (and nonanimal[40]) thought, memory, and sensitivity, and then finally connect the dots to form a pointillist (the points are back, finally doing something useful) picture of environmental nostalgia—this nostalgia of nonhuman assemblages. To get there, though, requires reading Boym (despite her text) against Illbruck to forge the first link in the cart's chain between (not a given) memory and nostalgia.

Illbruck writes, importantly, that in its early modern formulation as a disease, nostalgia had nothing to do with memory and everything to do with imagination—according to the first observers of nostalgia, there were no memories (or even sense memories) associated with the illness, state, or feeling, only hallucinations.[41] It is worth pausing, therefore, as historians, to ask when nostalgia became a problem of memory (if it ever did), rather than, or in addition to, imagination. Illbruck's study does a brilliant job of tracing these (partial) transformations—but, sadly, for us, it is another field with a no trespassing sign posted against it. We do, though, need to point to the field and recognize its presence, because if this work were a study of nostalgia in and of itself (rather than variations on a type of thought or existence, a set of feelings or ways of living, that have come to be termed "nostalgia") it would be irresponsible to jump, blindly, from the thing that is nostalgia to the thing that is memory and back again.

Given present methodological conditions, though, go ahead and jump. Boym, as a nice springboard, for example, laces together in a beautiful and elegant way—beyond what we've already seen—the classical Greek "art of memory" and the nostalgia of place or space that is the topic, *topos*, of her book. "According to legend," she writes, a poet protected by Castor and Pollux was saved from a roof collapsing over the house in which he had just been singing lyric hymns, and he was able, as a survivor, to identify the dead victims by where the guests had been sitting. "A miraculous survivor of the disaster," Boym glosses this story, he thereby "discovered the techniques of memory used by ancient orators, connecting places in the familiar environment (physical *topoi*) to stories and parts of discourse (rhetorical *topoi*)."[42] The graceful efficacy of this analysis as an ingress into a conversation about nonhuman memory as nonhuman nostalgia makes up for the fact that whereas "topography" and "Mnemosyne" would undoubtedly pass the angry Classics scholars test, "nostalgia" would fail horribly. It doesn't matter. The Classics scholars can go commiserate with the ironic modernist architects in the corner.

After all, scholars of rhetoric and communication, if not necessarily Classicists, have long claimed that rhetorical memory—this memory that (verbal and moving though it may be) is more often than not responsible for flushing out that slippery, non-verbal or never easily verbal thing, nostalgia—is (and has always been) other than purely human, subjective, or cognitive. Jeff Pruchnic and Kim Lacey, for example—against Boym, and giving hope to the replicants (but likely annoying the Classicists yet again)—have shoved ancient philosophers and rhetoricians together with technological systems, networks, and intelligences by arguing that the computational memory of today's information technology strongly resembles "the non-cognitive and asignifying" rhetorical memory (or "*mnemosyne*") described by the "early Greeks."[43] Both contemporary and very early Greek memory, in other words, are in Pruchnic's and Lacey's scholarship, affective, organic, mechanical, and material rather than cognitive or subjective.[44] Both types of memory separate the activity that is remembering from mind or communicative language, and neither privileges subjective experience over material operation.[45]

Moreover, the "ability to 'forget' the content of experiential memory" is, for Pruchnic and Lacey, a key component of both classical and contemporary memory processing. Memory, as a rhetorical operation, as music played and then echoing, never mourns the lost narrative, the misplaced experience, or the coherent initiating event that, supposedly, kick started the program or the physical operation in the beginning. On the contrary, forgetting, losing content, invoking hallucinatory, half-felt sensations, they argue, is a necessary prerequisite to remembering through "our bodies' affective responses," through "information networks,"[46] or, obviously, via trigger happy nostalgia. Collections of particular, physical, decontextualized experiential objects fail to hit coherent content-based narrative— and that is how rhetorical memory, memory processing, is, they imply, supposed to work.

Emphasizing the importance of physical "program" over subjective experience in early Greek as well as contemporary computational memory, Pruchnic and Lacey thus demonstrate that memory as a process has, and has had, value that memory content lost, if it ever had it to begin with.[47] Computational remembering, nonhuman memory, the memory of technological assemblages, according to this long term—if broad brush strokes—historical analysis, predates by centuries digital computers and digital technology. Swimming, submerged, in the primordial ooze, in the primeval puddle is not just nonhuman thought and memory, not just nonhuman (at least, it seems) nostalgia, but, narrowly, computational, technological, and rhetorical thought, memory, and nostalgia.

Even so, Pruchnic and Lacey shy away from the ooze and the puddle in their study, focusing their discussion of this non-cognitive rhetorical memory instead on human minds, human affect, and human bodies. Even as they demonstrate memory creep—the encroaching, itself remembering, slime and debris that afflicts, and transforms, Boym's urban topographies—even as they describe the gradual extension of memory beyond bodily borders, beyond communication and human language, across physical assemblages and accumulations, their interest remains the instrumental purposes that memory might serve for humans. In describing the spatial attributes of both classical and contemporary memory programs, for example, Pruchnic and Lacey ask us to consider, in a far less evocative, nostalgic sort of way than Boym's comment on the same moment,

> one of the most popular [early] memory techniques, the method of *loci,* in which parts of speeches or arguments were mentally associated with elements in an imagined physical location such as a house. As a technique, the method of *loci* is almost wholly a program; though there are many variations on this program, and an unlimited number of items or associations that might be worked within the program, the "content" of the technique is composed only of the act of association (between mental ideas and physical locations) itself.[48]

Rather than dwelling on the nostalgic qualities of the houses that are not only remembered, but themselves, memory, however, Pruchnic and Lacey instead describe the "diagrammatic" potential of such memory networks— in particular their relationship to "the material and electronic networks of information technology and the affective and biological economy of the nervous system."[49]

In this way, unlike Boym with her places (houses or cities) full of uniquely human affect, irony, and sensory stimulation, Pruchnic and Lacey, with their house as diagram, make room for computers and machines.[50] The memory network as house or place, they state, *is* computational in that it is "a program," in that it is characterized by process rather than content, and in that it extends beyond a purely linguistic human brain. Perhaps more haunting, this program involves not simply emptying memory of content in the name of process, and not just privileging the shudder or the satisfaction of repeated encounters, in various rooms, over the cognitive pleasure of a single moment of recognition in, say, the entryway, but also deliberately smearing the topography, the domestic space, the house, the swamp that gives rise to *nostos* with the same physical sensory memories that left their adhesive trail across Boym's urban landscapes. This memory technique is undoubtedly computational, in other words; but one might just as easily call it bacterial. And it is wantonly nostalgic.

Pruchnic and Lacey, however, do not take their argument into this smeary realm—their diagrams are crisp and clear. Like Boym's, in fact, the rooms that Pruchnic and Lacey set aside for the machines and information processing systems are small and constrained (although, not to worry— infinity can be microscopic as well as the size of a house). These memory programs are, in short, according to their analysis, tools—valuable only in that they assist humans in their quest to remember. Pruchnic's and Lacey's description of memory programs, inverting and twisting in on itself, then, eventually discounts, it seems, the possibility that memory might be divorced from human interactions. They imply that the activity of remembering—even if it is externalized, or perhaps especially if it is externalized—can be only a human activity. They leave the conventional roles that "cognition" and "mind" have played in the "extended cognition" or "extended mind" models on which they draw in the antechamber of the bad Descartes, prior to his reinvigoration, always aiming toward bounded, coherent, modern human-style consciousness.

But what if we take rhetorical memory seriously as a nonhuman— computational, mechanical, digital, or throw in bacterial as well—process? What if we push Pruchnic's and Lacey's claims together with Boym's nostalgic *topoi*? One potential implication is that memory, nostalgia, of this sort might produce a wholly computational (or bacterial) world. If the *loci* method works properly—not necessarily as a backdrop, screen, scrim, diagram, or set of connections—the *loci* or the *topoi* (choose your dead civilization), become, themselves, memory, computational, bacterial, or otherwise. They become not just an information processing tool, but a type of thought in and of themselves that, via infinite iteration and processing, achieves the creepy thrill that nostalgia initially promised only to homesick Swiss soldiers on the verge of modernity.

This idea—that computers or algorithms, themselves, think and become thought, beyond the realm of instrumentality—is no newer to scholarship than the notion, noted, that rhetorical memory remains relevant to more than purely human subjects. Luciana Parisi and Stamatia Portanova, for example, in the midst of their (likewise neurosis-inducing—neither the dining table nor early posthumanist scholarship is safe) critique of extended mind and distributed cognition models, define memory, and especially the affect leaking out of memory, as a specifically computational and mechanical rather, than cognitive (again in the bad Descartes sort of way) mode of thought:

> Whilst we do share with the "extended mind" hypothesis the idea that thought is not limited to the biological skin, we reject the syntax model of thought and the connectionist ontology on which it is grounded. Why should digital algorithmic processing be just another instance of a universal and predetermined grammar of thought? ... can there ever be new modes of thought that can escape this "mind" model?[51]

In asking these questions, Parisi and Portanova condemn what had once seemed a useful alternative to that pernicious, self-contained, deathless Cartesian subject. The extended mind model, they state, simply hammers this subject back together again with, granted, some attractive steampunk type bolts. Doing away with the skin or turning the machine or environment into a "prosthesis,"[52] after all, does not alter the basic definition of "thought" as human cognition that works on or via matter. If anything—working tirelessly through its distribution and extension—this model exposes all matter or all machines to continued colonization by Cartesian cognition (not to mention bad, not recuperated Darwinian hierarchies).

To challenge the idea that the machine merely "complement[s] human thought," or that "machines are just another instance of a mindware operating a hardware,"[53] therefore, Parisi and Portanova write that "the machine is its own thought, without having a supplementary dimension that grounds its cognitive structure."[54] The machine is for them not a tool or appendage—and computation is not a variation on human expression or human communication. Indeed, computational thought is contained rather than extended in their work—like nostalgia, it is cemented into place. Here, though, thought and memory are contained within a digital environment, within a field of signals that shift, appear, and reappear, rather than within an organic body, a Cartesian mind, or a bounded, visualizable space. The problem with Cartesian models of thought, according to Parisi and Portanova, is not that these models ignore all matter beyond the human brain; it is that they place the brain into a necessary relationship with all matter.

Where, then, does this leave rhetorical memory as nonhuman (computational, bacterial, or otherwise) memory? In Parisi's and Portanova's universe, it bolts it (using a different hammer) to machines or to algorithms that are, themselves, memory. Alongside Boym's city (and wrecked house) that is memory, Pruchnic and Lacey's pure and diagrammatic (yet hauntingly open to infinite exploration) domestic space that is memory, add, gingerly, carefully, now Parisi's and Portanova's field of fluttering, fluctuating digital shifts and signals—not to mention, of course, Chrostowska's messy archive of hoarded, replicating data that is memory (for itself—because no one else is looking) and Baudrillard's furniture stores full of exasperated gods that are memory. In each of these descriptions of the memory that concerns us, that provokes the rhetorical jump or the nostalgic shudder, human consciousness (it goes without saying—communicative speech being something of a non-starter when the subject dissipates) and cognition situated in the brain have fallen by the wayside. Like biopolitical reproduction, the memory that counts keeps leaning, ever closer to, invading the space of, the nonhuman assemblage.

Likewise, in each of these descriptions, memory is environmental—the infinite particularity and compulsive repetition that make remembering in this way so pleasurable are not purely linguistic; they infect and transform places, spaces, and fields (and, obviously, forests) into sensitivities and thus, themselves, memory. The magic of this mode of memory is its transformation of an atmosphere (to misunderstand Baudrillard)—say a forest, a house, or an expanding collection of sliced up embryos—into, itself, thinking data and matter. Nostalgia does its saccharine work (saccharine being a great favorite of the inhabitants of petri dishes) not just by playing merry hell with time, the abstract, and the particular, not just by turning constant repetition, the constant re-experiencing of an initial event that may never have happened, into something infinitely desirable, but also by leaving detritus and debris all over the environments it encounters, changing, irrevocably the work of these places.

And so, to regroup: we have now collected ourselves—and even, against our better judgment, collated—a series of defining characteristics of nostalgia and of memory *as* nostalgia. We've also pinpointed, using the pins for better purposes, the points and places at which this nostalgia and memory seem not to adhere to a purely human model. One experiment that remains unfinished, though, is watching nostalgia, so defined, come up against more mainstream scientific writing on nonhuman thought and sensitivity. The bacteria have been clamoring outside the walls of this chapter, even pushing themselves in through the cracks and chinks on occasion, muddying up, for example, the gears of the machines and replicants that had just, two and six paragraphs up, made it out of the storage spaces into which they'd earlier been consigned. It's time to give them their due.

The sensitivity and memory of organic systems—call these systems a single cell or an aggregate of living material such as bacteria or slime mold—have been popular players in scientific papers for a number of decades now. There are hundreds[55] of studies of bacterial memory and amoebic sensitivity circulating and flowing throughout scholarly databases, most premised on the simple notion that organic material, writ large, thinks.

Many of these studies also set aside—as irrelevant rather than politically interesting—nineteenth- and early-twentieth-century narratives of flattering hierarchical steps from simpler (cyanobacteria) to more complex (human) organisms. The thought, memory, and sensitivity of organic systems as systems—and as confusingly computational systems, more often than not—slips into dust and sand when faced with "our closest relatives, the great apes" type talk. Memory mocks close linear relationships—even in *Nature* and *Cell*.

In his book, *Wetware*, for example, the biologist Dennis Bray makes a case for the simultaneously organic and cybernetic qualities of cellular sensitivity and memory. He does so, first of all, by repeatedly, even compulsively, reminding his readers that the cellular thought he is describing is not the same as awareness or self-consciousness; it is not human thought.[56] No need to worry about making such a mistake now, however—the trauma of Cartesian self-consciousness is still with us; no one wants to trigger it again in an investigation of nonhuman nostalgia.

Second, therefore, and more interesting, he also (and also repeatedly) highlights two aspects of cellular thought—memory and sensitivity (or memory as sensitivity)—as the key, defining aspects of incipient organic thought, if not self-knowledge. With reference to the first, he states that "biological systems," "captur[e] a picture of their surroundings in molecular terms," and thereby "acquire knowledge of the world in a way no other chemical or physical system can."[57] Although resembling the "storage of memories by higher animals," however, the memory of, say, a bacterial system is "highly predictable and stereotypical," less "dependent upon the training regime and the internal psychological state of the organism."[58] Some might read this characterization of bacterial memory as an undesirable cognitive state—but hold off on judgment. Bacteria, after all, remember in this scenario, whereas higher organisms translate memory into narrative and abstraction. More on that soon—let's turn now to his second interest, sensitivity.

In another set of passages, Bray writes that "living cells have an intrinsic sensitivity to their environment—a reflexivity, a capacity to detect and record salient features of their surroundings—that is essential for their survival. I believe these features to be deeply woven into the molecular fabric of living cells."[59] Like bacterial memory, in other words, cellular sensitivity as it is described here is pure sensitivity, unadulterated by narrative. And so, mysteriously, when he puts the memory of bacteria together with the sensitivity of the cell, the resulting soupy, bubbling stew should look (smell, feel, sound—there's that echo again) familiar. Describing "the images"—are they projected onto a screen?—that are "captured by the cell," indeed, he states that they

> include everything from recent events to the distant past, rather like a picture taken on a family vacation. In the foreground are the fluxes of ions and small molecules that capture the moment . . . [I]n the middle distance, protein molecules display evidence of the recent past encountered by the cell in their states of chemical modification and conformational shape . . . [I]n the background of the composition we have the genetically specified chemical terrain shaped over millennia by evolution—sequences in DNA and structures of proteins that have remained virtually unchanged . . . a living cell contains an image of the world because it is born of the world.[60]

So is this external memory? Distributed cognition? Data processing? It's hard to tell when there is no gap at all between the matter and information that are remembering, thinking, storing, sensing, or feeling and the space, place, house, petri dish, dirt, field, *loci*, or *topoi* that are being remembered, thought, stored, sensed, and felt. And don't forget the evocative, echoing collision of the recent past and distant millennia, all cozily framed in the photo from the family vacation. In sepia tones, perhaps? "Nostalgia" comes to mind—creeping out of the corner like it always does—as a, perhaps, more accurate term.

Where Bray sees cellular memory as molecular transformation, after all, Crinson, Boym, Pruchnic, Lacey, Parisi, and Portanova might see it as the material or digital transformation of field, forest, house, city, or environment into memory—they might recognize, ricocheting around the embryo room, the nostalgic slime that transforms *topoi* and *loci* into, themselves, experiential and discursive databases. Or, whereas Bray might differentiate the predictable and stereotypical memory storage of bacteria from the psychological self-narrative of higher organisms, Chrostowska, Baudrillard, and Illbruck might call him up short and register doubt. They might cite the insistent, repetitive, predictable, and implicitly dysfunctional compulsions of higher organisms as well, falling flat while reaching, futilely, for the supposed psychological self, and then turning, always, predictably to the affective and physical stereotype and stutter—bad when it is trauma, and, well, also bad but secretly pleasurable and satisfying when it is a nostalgic revel and romp through the impossible infinity of a few favorite objects bloodying up the abstract narrative.

Finally, where Bray might posit the vacation photo metaphor as an effective rhetorical move because cellular memory is so evidently different from vacation shots, Braidotti might see in the two a sinister similarity, and thus a potential, less sinister, for the politically productive construction of nonhuman nostalgia (or even utopia)—for finding all the time in the world. The cellular holiday snap, you see, is utopian, necessarily no place, because it is intuited, detected, felt, and then recorded across a morphing, mutating set of living, dying, replicating proteins and molecules. The place, the thing, and the thought are all on top of one another. Likewise, it is nostalgic because, and one does need to acknowledge the violence of it here, it leaves the future, or futures, fragile and vulnerable to insults as well as assaults from a nearly infinite, yet only half remembered, and of course hardly experienced past—the past of millennia, of the sensitivities of ancestors and environments so long dead that they can be felt only as they creep across and colonize the cellular future.

But, violent though it can be, this nostalgic torturing of time—and then taking a faded snapshot of it—is also a far cry from the Kantian targeting (and killing, and mounting) of an ideal future (hanging, suspended, painfully, next to equally dead lost time). At least in the swamp of primordial nonhuman nostalgia, the future just gets a bit bruised. And it remains vital, once more, because in this swamp, shot through with nostalgia, politics is not only not transcendental, it is embedded in time *as* matter—in the twisted, inverted temporal physicality that is quite natural, and in fact disgracefully cozy, to bacteria and other nonhuman assemblages, but only available as a distant, faint, blurry copy. Like the half-seen echo, if you concentrate, cognitively, Cartesianly, on nostalgia, it dissipates. Like the ghost that the reverberation of the smell of the formaldehyde that once preserved the sliced up embryos whistles up, if you look directly at it— with that visual sense so dear to those invested in lines and linearity— it disappears. But it leaves you something, that hollow, thudding, pain, as it departs—and hence you know that it has force, and, importantly, political value.

Readers, hopefully, will thus finish this chapter, first, with a discordant, irritating ringing and reverberation in their ears—redolent of drunk, departed musicians, tangled, snarled tapestries, and ghostly slices of embryonic matter, behind glass—and second, more important, with a likewise irritating sense that the feeling that this sensory detritus stirs up, nostalgia, is more politically viable than even its embarrassed, awkward apologists have already, half-heartedly suggested it is. Nostalgia has become something of a cottage industry over the past decade or so—a cottage industry, undoubtedly, with an authentic working water wheel and artfully distressed wooden joints holding up the carefully treated straw roof. This industry has been driven, though—if obliquely, via breezes from different quarters—by the resurgence of humanity as an appropriate topic of humanistic inquiry, and by the fading fashion of the nonhuman and posthuman as categories of analysis.

But having already harped on the fact that the politics of life, biopolitics, is not only open to posthuman or nonhuman interpretation, but necessarily, always, inexorably trending toward nonhuman democracy, why not make the same insistent case about a more focused, pointed (pierced now) political problem: nostalgia? The reproduction and thought that erupt out of nonhuman biopolitics—once accepted as such—are disturbingly close to the repetition and memory (or, with thanks to Illbruck's early modern physicians, imagination) that keep attaching themselves to nostalgia. If there is a single lesson to be learned from this chapter, therefore, it is that nostalgia has political legs, cilia, but only as a nonhuman mode of thought (not to mention reproduction). Human nostalgia falls flat.

And this is not the case just because of all of the posthuman things that continue to populate the political scene, despite their waning trendiness— the autopoetic databases of stored family photos and memories (real ones, this time—not Bray's cellular metaphor), the ignored gods hanging around in bourgeois dining rooms planning the destruction of ancient monuments, the cars eating up time while the watches, via GPS, eat up roads, the brand new haunted houses planned by mid-century developers, the cities smeared with debris living a life of its own, or the stripped and strip-mined reproductive matter making up the chilly, empty Blechschmidt collection. In addition, it is because only assemblages absent a sense of self and other, absent a search for narrative, absent cognition in the bad-Descartes sense of the term can enjoy—absent even guilt now—the temporal matter or material time, the physicality of a past that constantly wounds, but never kills, the future. The endless repetition in the gap between the particular and the abstract can bring enormous satisfaction—and has enormous democratic potential. But there is also quite a hefty price tag attached to it—or, floating around, detached, within it. It is a gap, after all—replete with blinding reverberations.

Embryos

Remember, before, the faint feel of emergent ghosts summoned up in the chilly post-party emptiness of the echoing model room? Those ghosts will take center stage in this chapter's case study, the first of two, of the nonhuman nostalgia underlying ongoing biopolitics. Or, at least, psychic medium style, hints and traces of these ghosts will clatter and tap their way around the following pages, likely annoying the reader with their kitschy persistence. But irritation can be valuable—sometimes more so than a nobler emotion. Irritation sticks in the mind and raises small welts on the skin. And if it is not hauntingly nostalgic, helpful to humans, at the very least it can aggravate a human reader into considering a scholarly topic, *topos*—bits of nostalgic embryonic matter, slime, as the biopolitical norm—that a smoother, less tiresome style might not. This is something that chintzy late Victorians knew quite well.

The chamber starts out, however, spare. Recently cleaned, vacuumed, and disinfected, the model room has the cold, sharp clarity of ice on a midwinter night. But as the ice is sliced into ever thinner sheets of embryonic material, reproductive matter, placed behind plastic and glass, this clarity shivers and distorts. The echo of the music gives way to a group of murmuring, not quite decipherable, phantom voices; and the tangled, woven threads and strings from the partially unraveled ancient Greek tapestry begin to swing, faintly, in a way that the nonexistent breeze in the empty room fails to explain. The embryonic matter thus has an afterlife, a ghostly imprint, an unexplained face-like smudge looking out of the far corner window of an old photograph—but this afterlife is also (and here is the strident, scholarly point) a useful norm, a model, among models, of modern political life. The embryonic slime, because of its ghostly refusal to go away, because of its eerie replication in sound, smell, taste, and raised hackles, is a perfect example—though one of many—of a biopolitical figure whose reproductive life is also nostalgic life. So the argument in this chapter is trifold—and it will be repeated, endlessly, irritatingly: embryonic slime is a biopolitical norm; the reproduction of embryonic slime (not—don't be confused—embryos as products of reproduction) is thought; this reproductive thought, in turn, is, narrowly, nostalgia. (Corollary: and hence it packs its political punch).

There are other, more prominent, ghosts populating this chapter as well—one might imagine a cobwebbed corridor lined with gilt framed portraits complete with terrifyingly mobile eyes. These ghosts, however, are the eighteenth-, nineteenth-, and early-twentieth-century scientists, embryologists, and natural historians whose writing, variously, forms the primordial, mixed up glop out of which the samples of embryonic slime will coalesce and present themselves as thinking, nostalgic biopolitical life, hovering momentarily above the surface, before collapsing and flopping back into the murky fluid. A proper historian, it is true, would also carefully contextualize each of these damp writers within some sort of milieu (political, social, economic, legal, cultural, agricultural, take your pick) and then explain how the biopolitical life and thought each conjures up reflects and influences x, y, or z context—another endless, repetitive, circular, yet oddly satisfying task. And indeed, a distinct taxonomic temptation—especially given the nicely spaced intervals separating each of the haunted portraits—beckons here, to present this chapter, in its entirety, as an extended list: Entry 1: biography, context, text, life, oozing bit of thought and matter whose phantom presence undermines completely . . . Entry 2: biography, context, text, life, etc.

Perhaps taxonomic precision is not the best approach. True, there are organizing principles systematizing these texts—each of these writers enjoys embryos, and each makes coy remarks about the political life, thought, and nostalgia of embryonic material as reproductive, reproducing, replicating matter. But, to remain in keeping with Chrostowska's and Baudrillard's well-taken arguments, these organizing principals, satisfying though they may be, are, despite themselves, completely irrelevant to the collection and effective (or evocative) presentation of particular texts of this sort. Go do a search on Google Books for "embryos"; if categorically precise historical method still seems like a good idea, then initiate your own taxonomy—and enjoy your well-spent life. Here, however, rather than imagining a wall of well-spaced, madly grinning, chattering, carefully framed portraits vanishing into the dim, haunted distance, think instead of a splintered wooden box, full of chips of paint, crumbling vellum, strips of canvas, and thin strips of what used to be gilt, shoved to the back of a drawer in a cupboard that was just taken out of a storage facility. Same matter, same portraits—but much more conducive to interacting, mingling, chemically reacting with the equally ghostly bits and pieces and chips of embryos that are likewise eager to be read in this chapter.

As a concession to the anxieties of proper historians, though, here, after all, is a quick, slick list of the writers who will move glasses, ring bells, knock five times, and mess with the electricity over the course of this chapter: Georges-Louis Leclerc Buffon (1707–1788), Jean Baptiste Demangeon (1764–1844), Auguste Duméril (1812–1870), Félix Hement (1827–1891), William Thierry Preyer (1841–1897), Pierre Flourens (1794–1867), Charles Sedgwick Minot (1852–1914), and Bahaeddin Şakir (1874–1922). And, to flesh them out a little bit, before dissolving them back into smears of paint, swirling into the goo, here also are some biographical tidbits to pin to them

(and then watch the pins clatter back down to the ground). Buffon, cura-
tor of the Jardin du Roi, wrote copiously on natural history, mathematics, rhetoric, race, female semen,[1] and the saving majesty of the moose as
an example of a strong American quadruped.[2] Demangeon, in addition to
writing a short, spare work on semen, salt, and nervous fluid, got himself
expelled from university in Leipzig for being a "Jacobin."[3]

Auguste Duméril, zoologist, and Professor of Frogs and Fish, died, vio-
lently, in 1870, not from an amphibious toxin or a fishy spine, but from
yet more revolutionary activity during the Siege of Paris.[4] Félix Hément,
inspector of schools, writer of popular scientific works, pre-figuring by
a good century the spate of talking, cooperating, tolerant, educational
dinosaurs and anthropomorphic germs fighting anthropomorphic white
blood cells that teach today's school children the importance of being
human, also took a stab at defining "liberty of conscience" with reference
to biological development.[5] William Thierry Preyer, born in England,
writing in German, translated into French, physiologist, child psycholo-
gist, and more than a little interested in the rappings and tappings that we
keep hearing out of the corner of our ear in this chapter, was a humanist
with a remarkably healthy—or is it unhealthy? Slippery term—fascination
with anencephalic fetuses. He liked them. A lot.[6] Pierre Flourens (scoot
back a few decades here—it makes sense when you get to the next part
of the chapter) was a pioneer (see Buffon's moose and his eventual, reluc-
tant acceptance of American hardiness) in the field of experimental neuroscience, helped to develop anesthetic as it is used today, and was well
respected enough at his death to decompose in the vicinity of Georges
Ocurat and Marietta Alboni in Père-Lachaise cemetery.[7]

Minot, an anatomist, founder of the American Society for Psychical
Research, collector, himself, of a not unremarkable collection (around
1,200) embryos in his own right, was born and died in Massachusetts—
and also lived and worked there (*The Problem of Age, Growth, and Death*
not so much of a problem when tied, permanently with New England
tenacity, to the same cold, muffled acres—hard to transport the embryo
collection anyway).[8] One wishes there were something "Jacobin" about
him—but no. Finally, Şakir, a true mismatch to staid Minot (so staid, he's

equally freakish), was a late Ottoman statesman, dead before the declaration of the Turkish Republic, a physician, a founding Young Turk member of the Committee of Union and Progress, more likely than not an engineer of the Armenian Genocide (see his early-ish death, before the failed postwar trials), and thus, in addition to a scholar of embryonic development and decomposition, a war criminal.[9] He was not a humanist. And yet, like Preyer, he also, as we will see, very much liked his anencephalic fetuses.

Hopefully this schematic scattering of bits of biography will satisfy readers inclined to human interest sufficiently to trick them into considering, also, how the nonhuman or not quite human reproductive matter these figures studied and described flourished and replicated in politically resonant ways. These readers might start to wonder how this reproductive matter was thinking, contemplating, and nostalgically transforming itself and its environments into memories that satisfied because they repeated, endlessly, in the gap between the infinitely particular and the infinitely abstract. For example, Buffon's proto-evolutionary take—artfully forgotten, oops, by an early Darwin[10]—on organic (as well as inorganic, and oddly—see Pruchnic and Lacey—computational) life and thought as products of dynamic fields and systems, draws on animal, vegetable, and even mineral development to tell a story of life, reproduction, and embryonic development that is contingent and incomplete, always embedded, leaking out into, and becoming a story of thought, politics, and environment.

Prefiguring Leuckart's melancholy inability to fit parts together into wholes—or to imagine wholes in any form—Buffon writes that although embryonic life works and organizes itself, it can never achieve a distinct identity as a whole *or* a part; it thinks in a manner at odds with the absolute ideal to which it ostensibly aspires.[11] Buffon in this way defines life and reproduction as thought and growth—but as unusual, eccentric varieties of thought and growth that operate on their own terms. He compares, for example, cognition fevering the brain, to fertilization and embryonic development infecting, and heating up or energizing the womb, the body, and then multiple bodies and environments.[12] Thought, in his work, seeps into, infects, and then saturates living matter, while life becomes the stuff of perception, experience, and contemplation. Life becomes thought and reproduction becomes a thought operation in a way that only the nonhuman biopolitics of the previous chapters could have facilitated.

In making the case that viviparous organisms have eggs in the same way that oviparous organisms have, for example, Buffon writes that the womb conceives (organically and intellectually) the fetus via "a type of contagion that the male liquor communicates to it."[13] Magnets communicate magnetic qualities to iron; the "masculine contagion" infects the womb and then the entire female body;[14] the brain conceives ideas; and the womb conceives a fetus—or, the text twisting in on itself, just as "the ideas that the brain conceives are similar to the images of the objects it receives through the senses, the fetus, which is the idea of the womb, resembles that which produces it."[15] Fertilization, growth, and development, past, present, and future, perception, thought, and experience thus all infect and interpenetrate one another in this reproductive environment—emitting an embryonic mist that smacks of atmospheric affect rather than linear genetic transfer. Meanwhile, sperm, although "organized bodies," are better described as "natural machines than as animals,"[16] moving throughout this reproductive fog like artificial automatons rather than like organisms, without rest,[17] and without "will."[18]

Buffon, that is to say, has no patience for arbitrary distinctions between the conception of perceptions, of memories, of awareness, of affect, of appreciation, and the conception of matter, of what would come to be called genetic information, of bodies, of flesh, and of fluid (is the fluid nostalgic, political, or organic? The distinctions are irrelevant). "Contagion," as the best description of embryonic life, thought, reproduction, replication, and memory—or, as Luciana Parisi has posited it, as the best description of affective algorithmic thought, architecture, and intuition[19]—shoves into ever closer quarters biological life, growth, and reproduction and sensory, affective, intellectual life, growth, and reproduction. Biological conception is an intellectual activity in Buffon's (not to mention Parisi's) writing, and nonhuman reproduction, the reproduction of matter, air, dust, and fluid, is, in an emergent sense, biopolitical. Conceiving ideas and conceiving organic atmospheres are the same process. Or, to try one more whack of this now, undoubtedly, repetitive and annoying hammer, living, thinking, reproducing, and perceiving, as environmental activities, cannot be dissociated from one another.

But don't forget: the contagion that is thinking, feeling, sensing, perceiving, or remembering life is also wrapped up in the communication of attractive qualities from mineral to mineral—and sperm, the organisms that seem most bent on an endpoint or goal, are aimless primarily because they are, like machines, without rest and unaffected, unaffective. In short, therefore (don't worry, we'll delve further into Buffon's "encyclopedic" inquiries in a bit), organic conception radiates a strain of thought that is indistinguishable from matter. It turns physical and intellectual environments into physically intellectual environments given over to remembered perceptions, it emits objects and ideas that are relational rather than absolute—the oozing output of matter interacting with matter—and it seems, inevitably, to be bent on missing its abstract goal.

Sperm, contrarily, and surprisingly marginal to Buffon's reproductive contagions, are more mechanical than organic, elements of the environment rather than initiators of a distinct, finite, proto-genetic progression. Endless, and endlessly particular, without rest, the thought activity of potentially reproductive sperm—it doesn't really make a difference, in Buffon's account, whether or not one lucky sperm, *Miracle of Life* style, comes across an egg—continues processing without any intention of reaching an end. Wrecking, with abandon, therefore, the walls built up by earlier philosophers to separate organic, intellectual, mechanical, and computational (proto-computational, if not proto-genetic) systems—the thought that Buffon conceives is irrelevant to classic rational cognition, but oddly familiar to Boym's relentlessly political *topoi* and Pruchnic and Lacey's less adamant, but nonetheless still ideological, *loci*.

From embryonic development presented as visceral, fluid, gluey thought, smeared across wombs, bodies, and then systems, places, and environments, Buffon turns to an extended analysis of "reproduction in general," which he initiates with a sop to the classical philosophers who so bothered Leuckart: a comparison of the "perfection" of the germ of a plant to that of the fetus of an animal—with the latter differing from the former only in its greater development or complexity.[20] From there, though,

Buffon backs off of the perfection so central to classical politics, the gesture toward potential wholes, and he investigates, instead, the life and liveliness that are "physical properties" of all matter, regardless of how dissipated, incomplete, and intangible it is[21]—the motes of dust swirling up and dispersing and dirtying what would become biopolitical mass democracy. He writes, for example, that there is in nature "an infinite number of permanent organic elements, all of them alive," whose substance is the same as that of organized beings, just as there is an infinite number of "inanimate/crude ("brute") particles that resemble inanimate/crude ("brut") bodies."[22] Infinite, replicating, reproducing, narrowly boxed up, particularity is the stuff of both organic and inorganic existence.

How does Buffon, though, cope with the absence of any complete or completed object in this story? He seems, after all, far less bothered by it than many who wrote both before and after him; there must be some reason for his relative lack of anxiety. His response—satisfying, but politically suspect to those who doubt the value of nostalgic repetition—is to translate, repeatedly, the complete object into an archive of undifferentiated, ever tinier, particular parts. When one must "separate, break up, and dissolve a cube of sea salt to see, through crystallization, the small cubes of which it is made,"[23] and when one must also separate the elements of a polyp to recognize its achievement as a life form,[24] one must also, having done so, having recognized this tiny, fragile, life in its wholeness, forget it (as Pruchnic and Lacey write), fail to perceive it (as Illbruck's early modern neurological patients do), and re-remember it only through faulty affect (as Baudrillard's recent bourgeoises do)—given that what was, potentially "whole," is now a heap of microscopic bits—the whole collapsed into a box of paint chips, which are entire in their own way.[25]

Or, as he writes of this gratifyingly impossible, Sisyphean (or perhaps Promethean) task of missed perception, since all living beings, no matter how complex, are composed of "active" and "living" "molecules," then all animal and plant life might easily be redefined as the waste, refuse, emissions, or for that matter deaths, of these same "particular," discrete, "tiny lives."[26] The ache here, in other words, is not just welling up from the fact that you need to kill the organism to view its distinct parts, but from the far more horrifying fact that the death of the organism is irrelevant to its life; the life of the organism, or any organism, could just as easily be described as the stuff squirted out of the smaller and smaller things that may or may not have coalesced—or coalesce in the future—into the faulty whole. There is no tragic death of a noble being for the sake of knowledge in this story. The death of the whole is no different from the defecation of some tiny, microscopic part of it. Indeed, no one notices the organism, dead on the side of the road (or alive in the lab), because thought and life seep, constantly, out of the bits and pieces of organic and inorganic stuff assembled and disassembled over geologic, rather than biological, time. The big, bounded organism was a type of debris or defecation when it was living its complex life; and it is the same sort of debris or defecation when it is decomposing by the wayside.

This all seems a far cry from "reproduction in general." For Buffon, though, appreciating life, conceived in the same way as an experience tied to a memory and then evaporated into an undifferentiated fog, is a necessary prerequisite to approaching (and then missing) the reproduction or replication of this life. "Life," regardless of how organized or complex it may be, is the diffuse refuse of a system of disconnected bits of molecular "lives" that transform the environments around them into their thoughts and experiences. Moreover, "life," especially as it relates to reproduction, is as relevant to mineral existence as it is to plant or animal existence—one cannot properly describe animal life without likewise describing plant and mineral life. Even as he repeatedly stresses "nature's" organic rather than inorganic goal (that can never be reached), the open-ended, yet concrete quality of "life" writ large leads Buffon back to something that might be called inorganic vitality, to hoards of digitally stored images and memories, to life as thought, to the biopolitics of nostalgia. Readers must keep this inorganic vitality in feverish mind, he insists, when they turn to reproduction.

Reproduction is in this way, for Buffon, as it is for Leuckart, nearly impossible to peel away from any other organic, inorganic, intellectual, or sensory operation. "In nature," he writes (in the eighteenth century—it would be too eerie by far for him to be invoking these assemblages without the occasional foray into Enlightenment era certainties), the "abstract" never exists, everything operates in relation to everything else, and this relational quality of natural existence must infect all thought of, and work on, reproduction. Expanding on his theme—and taking a dawdling roundabout route to "reproduction," again, the ostensible topic of its own, separate chapter—specialized taxonomic theories are certainly satisfying, but a specialist can never actually be certain that one organism or collection of inorganic particles is more "composed" than any other.

On the contrary, he continues, organisms that may seem whole are actually porous, absent distinct borders, a dynamic result of the relations that exist among all material particles. Fitting them up with abstract, unifying narratives (here, of reproduction) is thus perfectly fine, but—hear the echo—misses the point of the infinite particularity that ostensibly produces (reproduces) these narratives. The taxonomic narrative is nothing more than an obeisance to incorrectly predetermined human ideas about what constitutes complexity or composition.[27] Nothing escapes the logic of the system (not even the dining table)—except, Buffon writes, everything, and everything that reproduces.

Although scholars choose to draw lines among animals, plants, and minerals, Buffon then drives his argument home—and although these same scholars, with reason, choose to rank organisms (and inorganic collections of particles) according to their greater or lesser adherence to an abstract model "animal," or abstract model "plant"—such division, he insists, is arbitrary. These "lines of separation," do not exist "in nature," he writes, with that nicely historicized certainty, even if they exist in human minds.[28] And so the "life" that is particularly relevant, or relevant in its particularity, to reproduction must be understood to operate with abandon across organic as well as inorganic environments. It is not situated in specific, complex, organized, biological bodies; and it is alien—not in a monstrously fecund, late-twentieth-century sci-fi sort of way, but in a post-Enlightenment alienation sort of way—to abstract, cognitive, human thought. The thought that goes along with reproductive life as it keeps mushrooming across Buffon's heavy, encyclopedic volumes, once again, is relational, concrete, and systemic. And if there is a feeling that goes along with this thought, it is the elation of replicating, ceaselessly, in the gap between the infinite particularity of the tiny, microscopic, ever divided "lives" that keep infecting Buffon's reproductive environments, and the narrative of the whole organism that fails, in every way, to reflect them.

Given this interpretation of life or liveliness as less the embodied result of a distinct act—reproduction—than as a set of environmental relations, Buffon posits furthermore that the *death* (this is still in the chapter on "reproduction") that is ordinarily held up as the antithesis to reproduction also eludes abstract narrative or categorization. He writes, for example, that there are beings that are not "plant," "animal," or "mineral"—beings that "infest" what are frequently the dead or dying bodies of these same plants, animals, and minerals—and that these beings are as much alive as the body they inhabit might or might not be.[29] It is important, Buffon continues, to examine, therefore, these "intermediate beings" of organized bodies that, without reproducing like animals and plants, nonetheless possess a type of life, replication, flourishing, and movement—beings that can enter into the "constitution" of other lives—because they represent a type of life that is, itself, simultaneously death, a variation on the debris theme from before.[30] Shake up the bits of plaster, paint, and slices of embryos in the badly buckled drawer, Buffon is saying, and watch what ghosts emerge.

If readers do examine such beings, in fact, Buffon assures them that they will conclude that reproduction and generation are nothing more than a change of form that arises from the coalescence of particles—while the "destruction" of the "organized being" happens via the division of these particles.[31] Although a scholar might—given the diffuse quality of "life" and the arbitrariness of abstract taxonomies—distinguish between "living matter" and "dead matter" rather than between "organized matter" and "crude/brute matter," even this division will quickly turn into a bog, puddle, or muddle. After all, Buffon concludes, the "principal substance" underlying the rocks, marble, sand, and dirt that one ordinarily describes as "brute/crude" is the debris or waste of dead animals and plants[32]— reproductive life in this way playing out across the nostalgic bit of rock inhabiting its geological time.

Underscore this claim: in the sea of his discussion of embryonic life as concrete and present rather than abstract and future, as an assemblage rather than as a bounded whole, and as present in inorganic "dead" things as it is in organic "lively" things, Buffon wants to float a conclusion about reproduction. Buffon batters his readers, at length, encyclopedically, with the claim that reproduction, including human reproduction, summons up, undifferentiated, matter, memories, particles, ideas, and organisms. Even the animal or human womb is better understood as an element dissolved into an intellectual and material environment than as a discrete fabricating part attached to a discrete fabricated body. The womb, for example, growing both in volume and mass during embryonic development," develops, according to Buffon, its own "type of life" or its own "vegetation or development."[33] It is "not simply a sack that is destined to receive semen and contain a fetus," it is "not simply an ordinary extension of the body"; rather, its development is as much a variation on intellectual and material generation as the development of the fetus itself, or of any other animal or plant.[34] In short, "this type of growth is a true development, an increase [accroissement]" that can happen "only via the intimate penetration of organic molecules that are analogous to the substance of this part."[35]

One obvious, if tangential, conclusion to draw from this analysis is that Buffon was unusual among his contemporaries (as well as among those who came before and after him) in that he was unconvinced that there was any difference between what males and females contributed to reproduction.[36] Deliberately challenging the classic model of an implicitly rational male life force that initiated implicitly irrational female growth, Buffon ignored rationality in his discussion of growing, thinking, life, and posited, for example, the existence of female semen that worked along with male semen in the conjuring up of the ideas and memories that were also developing reproductive and reproduced matter. Female semen, Buffon wrote, was visible, along with its male counterpart, under a microscope, and it was equally responsible for the disposal or dispersal of both life and thought across reproductive environmental systems.[37] But let's pause for a moment to chart the rhetorical path that Buffon followed to this conclusion.

In elaborating this theory of female semen, Buffon begins by creating a monstrous, but oddly inviting, amalgam of his analogy between the womb and the brain and his seemingly unrelated argument that both viviparous and oviparous animals begin with eggs.[38] Rather than going from there to, say, the metaphor of the idea fertilizing the egg,[39] however, Buffon lets that seemingly nicely tied up branch whap back into his readers' faces. "If all animals and plants contain an infinite number of living organic parts," Buffon explains, "one should find these same parts in their semen . . . and the animalcules that one sees in the semen of males are only these same living organic molecules, or at least they are the first reunion or assemblage of these molecules."[40] As a result, "female semen should contain, like that of the male, living organic molecules, similar to those of the male"— and "since living organic parts are common to animals and plants, one should also find them in the semen of plants."[41] Female semen is not waiting, patiently, for inspiration to strike; it is itself the evidence that all living environments are always reproductive—that all places, all *topoi* and *loci*, without exception, are clouded over with a generative atmosphere. The sci-fi monster, in other words, is back with a vengeance, in the form of a mist—nothing, and especially sperm, has any claim to a linear, causal will; everything instead is participating, cloud like, in the constant generation of life and thought.

To bring this theory of fertilization and reproduction across bodies, environments, atmospheres, and universes, across biological, geological, and political time to a meaningful conclusion, therefore, Buffon takes his interpretation of male and female semen as similar assemblages of living organic molecules in the direction of what, to him, is a more evocative story of the creation and growth of embryonic or fetal material. He writes that within these reproductive atmospheres and environments, male and female semen must, "via some mechanism," form itself into "many fetuses, some male and some female," which, in turn, coalesce according to the "molecules that represent the sexual parts," in separate "spheres of attraction," each distinct because each could have only one "center."[42] Following the moment at which the simultaneous work of male and female semen infuse a "female" reproductive field with a magnetic type of energy, that is to say, the embryonic material that operates across it coalesces into a number of fetuses that come together randomly, according to the centripetal force acting within each sphere of attraction. The end result may be (incidentally) separate, sexually defined bodies, but the reproductive process, according to Buffon, is a process in which an accumulation or field of infinite and infinitely tiny reproductive data points integrate, operate, coalesce, and—more importantly—disintegrate, disperse, and dissipate. Embryonic matter is reproductive as much because it disintegrates, into ever thinner slices, as because it coalesces into something recognizable (and representable).

But what does this whirlwind or cloud of reproductive, reproducing life have to do with thought—or nostalgia? Where are the chattering ghosts? To coax them out, we might quietly line up the primary players in his story of reproduction—while discarding those he also dismisses. First, the discards: keep in mind that Buffon, once again, is frankly questioning the validity of any theory of reproduction that takes the egg and sperm—and thus lineage (linearity, that is, past, present, and future)—as its touchstone. Yes, he writes, egg and sperm are part of the reproductive process. But more important to this process is the magnetized or infected womb-as-body-as-brain-as field or environment.

And so, in Buffon's story, the successfully reproductive actants are: lively molecules, generative atmospheres, ideas and memories conceived in the same fluid space as conceived matter, death and decomposition that are secretly reproduction, reproduction that is secretly waste and debris, and endless motes of particles, constantly rising up and resettling in unexpected absent patterns. Or, to reformulate this collection in different (if now repetitive) words: reproduction infects all living matter in Buffon's model. And information is contagious. As a result, there is no matter or information—even that which dissipates instead of coalescing—that can be termed unviable, or waste. Storage and dispersal are as vital to reproduction as any chance, haphazard product that may or may not integrate itself back into the living environment.

And so Buffon, in yet other words, is describing, then, a reproductive environment that produces matter and thought with equal abandon, that operates most effectively in the gap between an infinitely iterated collection of unrelated, minute particular lively objects and the failed abstract unity that is always straining to emerge from them, and, most importantly, that translates the material and informational waste emitted by this system into further memory, further objects and data to store, across environments that—because of this ongoing replication and storage—become magnetized, living, thinking, and remembering systems. Buffon's reproducing embryonic material that infects and pollutes likewise embryonic environments is living matter that, upon the slightest touch or contact, conjures up a living field, always spinning out and shooting off other bits of living matter and place. It is a prime example of the tight interlacing of reproduction and thought that characterizes nonhuman life. Embryos may, depending on your politics, represent in a light, liberal sort of way, a potential complete form, but in the present, they are their own odd never complete, and certainly never human, assemblages.

Eschewing Leuckart's melancholy, Buffon thus takes his readers on a tour, first of life in its particular parts, and then of life in its infinite parody of a whole, and then of life as an ongoing thinking system, and then of the reproduction of life as a specific sort of thought—memory and matter all leaking into one another—and then finally of the detritus of life, never dead (there are the angry ghosts), failing to coalesce, but nevertheless getting swept up into a heap in the corner of a storage facility, and there starting, once again, to ferment in a contagious condition, into thought. His used up embryonic molecules, failing to meet, rotting in the corner, are identical to the trash that nostalgically transforms Boym's buildings into a living city. His wombs are Chrostowska's unvisited archives and unviewed databases. His story gets at the obliteration of divisions between contemplation and reproduction, between information and generation, and thus between reproductive, generative systems and the faulty memories embedded in them. And his work of natural history is in this way also a political history of nonhuman reproductive nostalgia. He started, despite himself, and despite Darwin's remarkable lack of remark, a trend.

Follow this trend into the nineteenth century, nudging to the side, with one toe, the heap of replicating, flourishing embryonic dust still fermenting, remembering, and enjoying itself along the edge of the path. Here, in an era most inviting to ghostly visitation—the uncanny and unsettling settling comfortably, cozily into the dining rooms inhabited by frustrated gods and confused furniture—here, despite conventional post-1859 Darwin (or following Grosz's now demonstrably accurate counter-reading of post-1859 Darwin), Buffon's assemblages of undifferentiated organic and inorganic biopolitical life, his embryonic material that coalesces with equal abandon into conceived matter and conceived ideas, his magnetized environments and places that reproduce as they remember, take on even greater vitality. At the very beginning of the century, for example, in 1829, Demangeon argued in a comparative study of "generation," that embryonic development operated on the same spectrum as the aggregation of "metals, salts, [and] earth."[43] Biological and geological time, the reproduction of organic life and the coalescence of place, immediately, once again, infecting one another.

From there, he likewise compares "nervous fluid" to "spermatic fluid" (the stuff that conceives ideas, memories, and perceptions to the stuff that conceives life), noting that although they are not the same, both nonetheless "vivify," both produce heat, force, or liveliness, both give off "subtle effluvia," both can be phosphorescent (enlightened?), and, both balance one another: one fluid, he states, cannot be exhausted without exhausting the other, each is secreted from the same source, "infinitely," and the secretion of each—"sympathetic" with the other—proves that "the organs of the body are like cogs in a machine, in which one cannot be harmed without the rest going haywire."[44] The liveliness, fluids, machines, magnetism, growth, flourishing, fecundity, memory, thought, and sensitivity that make up Buffon's world are reassembled here, that is to say, into a subtly altered, but still recognizable, breathing, shuddering set of motley *topoi*.

Or, in more measured terms, the rules that govern organic life, for Demangeon, are also the rules that govern the life of metals and other minerals, and the living fluid that generates life (spermatic fluid) is inseparable from the equally living fluid that generates thought and feeling. But Demangeon makes a metaphor of this overlap, first, between organic and inorganic life, and second, between thought and life *not* by invoking mind, self, logic, or brain. Instead he invokes the barely controlled rotation of cogs in a machine, always about to "go haywire"—the mechanical equivalent of the neuralgic nostalgia sufferers spinning their imaginative wheels into achingly, deeply felt memory. Intellectual "generation" and material "generation" are one in this theory of life, just as they were in Buffon's natural history—and just as in Buffon's narrative, this circulating, intertwining, tangled interaction of reproduction and thought spin out a sea of crazy, barely contained intellectual ferment, an infinitely iterated archive of damaging, physical memories.

Moreover, like Buffon, Demangeon also hacks a cozy nook out of, into, his story of "generation," life, reproduction, and development, and then places within this nook a sharp-cornered, awkwardly shaped, spindly meditation on death. Distinctions between life and death, Demangeon continues, as well as distinctions between seemingly complex and seemingly simple organisms are difficult to maintain *especially* when describing reproduction. The life of most animals, he explains, requires a certain degree of humidity in the air, and indeed such humidity can revivify formerly dead organisms such as (zombie) flies or polyps. More to the point (injected now into a cold, dead corpse) the zombie phenomenon can also be "observed" in "more perfect animals, for example in humans."[45] As an example of such an occurrence, Demangeon cites previous researchers, who noted that "a pregnant woman can appear dead, but nonetheless live again" under properly humid environmental conditions, giving "indications of vitality" especially when undergoing an emergency caesarian section.[46]

This living death that takes reproduction as a touchstone thus explodes any lingering, craggy distinctions between organic and inorganic matter. Returning, as Buffon also did at this point in his argument, to scholarship on infinitely divisible particles, with their "distinct lives," and "their faculty for voluntary movement," to the fact that, as they accumulate, they produce "every part of the animal system, the bile, the blood, the flesh, and the bones," Demangeon likewise makes a key (familiar) claim on the subject of organic and inorganic reproduction, generation, growth, and death: these living, dynamic particles, according to contemporary experts, appear as much in dead plant matter and as much in inorganic matter as they do in living animal matter.[47] Indeed, as one "celebrated botanist" had recently proved, "inorganic bodies themselves are nothing more than aggregations of living atoms," proving in turn that "in a word, matter is living."[48] Even the molecules of dead plants "having been submerged in water . . . turn on their axes, turn on themselves, and change their positions," just as the molecules of "solid rocks," "metals," and "all inorganic substances" do.[49]

Demangeon, in other words, presents and resolves the same apparent series of rewarding contradictions that Buffon does. It is true that his fascination with reproduction has a creepy, clinical, scalpel-clattering nineteenth-century edge to it—smugly situated within its rhetoric of women's reproductive dead bodies exposed and regulated. It is likewise true that whereas Buffon dismembers the female body as part of the general dissolution of all living debris—the womb dissipated across sensitive, reproductive environments in the same way that all other bodily (and not bodily) matter eventually is—Demangeon presents to his cool readers the story of a pregnant woman actually being cut to pieces. But Demangeon's conclusions on life, reproduction, thought, sensitivity, and memory are, despite the horror show framework, nonetheless the same: the dismembered, reproductive living-dead body operates as such only within a complex, chaotic field of vitality that incorporates everything from lively molecules to desiccated flies to dissolving plants to polyps to rocks and metals. All matter, Demangeon writes, is living and "nervous." Reproduction is a story of generative matter and generative sensitivities mutually exhausting and reinvigorating one another. "Generation" gives way to thought, which in turn lends itself, once more, to a nonhuman biopolitics of living, organic and inorganic assemblages, which gives way finally to a reproductive activity predicated on the sensitive re-experience, the aching memory of, previous, unlived lives. Nostalgia ties his generative world together.

Skip ahead a little less than a decade, and dwell for a moment, on a series of descriptions of embryonic and fetal material, especially human embryonic and fetal material, transforming itself into variations on places,

spaces, fields, systems, environments, and—to enjoy that repetition—
topoi and *loci*. These examples will come fast and furious for a few pages,
and then we can return to how and where these reproductive environments spurt out small puffs and bursts of thought, perception, sensitivity,
and memory. In 1836, for example, Joseph François Louis Deschamps and
Pierre Flourens entered into the debate about whether embryos derived
from "a germ" that formed out of "magnetic fluid, crystallization, or ani-
mation," or whether the "formation and development of the germ" resulted
from an "agglomeration of pre-existing organic molecules,"[50] by playing
on the popular early-nineteenth-century theme (more organ grinder than
contrapuntal conceptual music)[51] that, as the human embryo develops, its
various stages, as well as the stages of its various organs, reflect "the permanent states, and even organs, of [less elevated] vertebrates and inverte-
brates," with, for example, fetuses briefly possessing, say, the appendices
of batrachians or the cartilage of fish.[52] Fetal development in variations on
these themes mirrors what had become an increasingly rigorous natural
taxonomic structure.

Closed taxonomies, again, are very satisfying. But this one, actually, is
secretly quite leaky, lacking altogether the walls, barriers, beginnings, and
endings of proper taxonomic fortresses, and stuck all over with dripping
gutters and puddles of indecipherable goo. Indeed, despite the teleology—
the smug and satisfied (although infinitely less chilling than Demangeon's)
story of little human bodies gradually hitting their benchmarks—there is
also in this tale, a lack of any certainty about where the fetus begins and
where it ends (if it can be said to begin or end anywhere). As one proponent
of the theory suggested, in fact, this oddly zoological (see H. G. Wells) take
on reproduction and development is a useful departure from the " 'teleo-
logical' physiology" that dominated conversation at the time.[53] After all,
it is not the whole body (mourned by Leuckart, ignored by Buffon, and
cut to bits by Demangeon) of the developing fetus that reaches successive
developmental milestones, but arbitrarily designated pieces of the fetal
body that reach these tilted stone markers. Different organs reflect the
organs of different animals at various, unexpected, moments in its march
toward perfection and completion, or replete abstract unity.

Flourens's and Deschamps's developing fetus, as developing life, in this way spreads out across a speciously taxonomic system, rather than climbing in a linear way up an obvious step-by-step taxonomic ladder. Moreover, as it grows, it pokes un-mendable holes and rents (pointed objects useful once more) in the idea of a discrete human perfection toward which all life is ostensibly moving—even while, simultaneously, it mischievously removes important rungs from the hierarchal taxonomy at the top of which this human organism ordinarily resides. Flourens's and Deschamps's fetus becomes an environment, an array, a set of nicely placed, disconnected animal parts that fail to exist in any obvious relation to one another—a collection of infinitely iterated particular objects with zero reference to a unified abstract narrative. It becomes an unvisited archive and un-accessed database.

One might in fact draw the conclusion from Deschamps's and Flourens's presentation of this common story of fetal development not that a completely formed human is an animal that is and must be, because of its early development, a willing and tolerant participant in a diverse, difficult, but fundamentally welcoming ecology and environment, but that the fetus and the environment, only tangentially related to something that may or may not be human, are always smeared all over one another— the fetus always reflecting a horizontal lack of temporal or physical relations, reflecting objects cluttering up a splintered box, popping up all over the awkward place in confused timelines, rather than reflecting a vertical hierarchy of increasingly complex, self-contained wholes. In short, reproduction is not, here, the initiation of embodied life, but the reorganization of an infinitely iterated, disorganized, collection of particular bits of matter and information into an evocative, haunting, lack of an image.

Or, to make this nostalgic claim in more tech-savvy terms, the open-ended embryonic, reproductive environment or system, this set of coalescing *loci* that evoke objects floating around, embarrassingly, in time, is an informational system or environment. Not only is reproduction best defined, according to these nineteenth-century studies, as a systemic process or function, it is also best defined as an informational process or function. In quick, data dump format: consider, for example, Duméril, citing E. R. A Serres, who insists that development is "centripetal," and always occurs as "messages" pass from "the periphery toward the center."[54] Or, next, turn to Hément, who describes the informational quality of the reproductive environment via an extended meditation on the difference between generation via asexual division and generation via the sexual fertilization of an egg.[55]

In fact, it might be worthwhile to retrieve the debris that is Hément's analysis of the cracked egg and savor it for a few more paragraphs, picking bits and pieces of sticky dust from its exterior. Starting, therefore, with a familiar, now late-nineteenth-century, point about how the egg is always pure potential—something that is simultaneously the "present" and the "future," something that both "is" and "should be,"[56]—Hément veers off into his own underbrush, pursuing a series of much less expected arguments. From pure potential, for example, Hément goes on to write that the egg is also a source of "vital power,"[57] the first step in appropriate generation,[58] and the "depository of the laws" that govern the attraction to it of "surrounding bodies" and their combinations and dissociations.[59]

The egg, in short, is not "simply the fortuitous result of an association of mineral elements,"[60] but a distinctively computational, "law-" or "code-" governed, information-based, dynamic depository—both an archive and a prime mover. In tipsy and temporal, rather than purely technological, terms, then, the egg is thus "the future" not because of its always potential, abstract, unattainable end, and not because it will become an organic whole (Leuckhart's hopes dashed again), but because it operates simultaneously as reservoir or store of power or information and as a depository of laws and instructions. It is the future because of its computational, algorithmic affect and process: its laws or instructions work through or on its store or reservoir to generate successive combinations and dissociations that in turn churn out memories and experiences across a reproductive environment. Hément, that is to say, narrows Buffon's, Demangeon's, Duméril's, and Flourens's reproductive environment as thinking system into a reproductive environment as informational system. The nostalgic *loci* are taking on Pruchnic's and Lacey's computational coloring.

Whereas Hément's foray into the field of sliced up eggs and embryos, never reproduced, but always reproducing, as environments, thoughts, memories, and matter, led him to a mill and store, and then, with a few quiet hints and wisps of sci-fi suggestion, to the monstrous, ever-growing data hoards of the late twentieth and early twenty-first centuries, Preyer foraged in the same field and came up, instead, with environmental intuition, sensitivity, and, with similar hints and suggestions (speculative fiction speculative in all sorts of different ways), the raps, taps, sighs, and whispers of ghosts in the corner of the room. The reproductive nostalgia of embryonic information collides here, in other words, with a slight squishing sound, with the reproductive nostalgia of embryonic intuition. Preyer, for example, played insistently on the theme of the brain's relative lack of importance to both developing life and the thought that characterizes this life. Departing from earlier writers by emphasizing the circulation of the blood, rather than "nervous fluid," as the embryo's originary bodily function,[61] Preyer nonetheless finds in this function the same thought, sensitivity, and memory that Demangeon and Duméril had found in the circulation of nervous and, or as, spermatic fluid.

Preyer initiates this analysis by commenting on the lack of "muscle fibers" and "nervous elements" in the early organization of the circulatory system. The first contractions of the heart, he writes, are of "extreme physiological importance" because they indicate an enormous amount of energy output when there is still no trace of muscles or nerves. The cells that constitute the heart move by themselves, a diffuse system, and have no connection to a centrally organized structure.[62] In fact, "it is notable," he continues, "that neither the *brain* nor the *spinal cord* is necessary to the movements of the heart," a point that can be proved both by examining embryonic specimens in a laboratory setting and by considering the life of infants born without brains or developed respiratory systems (his favorite point—sharp and nerve wracking, this one).[63] Preyer dwells at length on these pinned down anencephalic embryos, fetuses, and newborns— of particular interest to physiologists, he repeats, because they demonstrate the minimal importance of cerebral function to development and movement.[64] Most interesting, he invites his readers to discover, is the extent to which they can "*feel*" threats, or a lack of air or nutrition, despite their missing minds and selves.[65]

Preyer indeed presses home the problem of embryos feeling pain, failing or succeeding in sensing, sleeping, and waking. And repeatedly, with much precise re-iteration, lined up neatly, he writes that although embryonic matter can experience such states, they cannot, and need not, think rationally about them. The brain is irrelevant to an embryonic sensitivity to pain, he states.[66] It is also only partially relevant to embryonic sensitivity in general. And as proof of this claim, Preyer invokes that elusive, amygdalar sense of smell. Since olfactory hallucinations are rare (unlike visual hallucinations)—with hallucinations necessarily the projection of a brain—an embryo cannot, according to Preyer, smell. Moreover, not only can't embryonic material smell, neither can it remember smells (unlike, implicitly, sights).[67] And finally, almost as an afterthought, since a fetus has no sense of self (tied up in memory and smell)—in the way that a person with a working brain has—it also cannot sleep or to waken. It is in an intermediate, always quasi sleeping, state.[68]

In a box, then, tied up with a bow, Preyer argues that embryonic matter can feel pain, sense threats, and fear a loss of air or nutrition—but it can do so only as a dissipated, open ended, not centrally coordinated, and only partially perceptive system or environment. Remove the first paper layer of the box, however, and see (or smell) more: the interplay of scent, sight, sleep, and hallucination in the second two experiments that Preyer conducts leads him to conclude that embryos can neither smell nor be called "awake" because olfactory sensitivity and wakefulness require, first, the ability to remember in narrative form, and second, the ability to distinguish, psychologically, between self and environment or other. Sight and quasi-wakefulness (call it by its proper term: dreaming[69]), however, are different. These two modes do not, according to Preyer, demand any psychological or rational pre-requisites—and the evidence that Preyer marshals in support of this distinction is the well-documented existence of visual (but not olfactory) hallucinations. Embryos without brains and narrative memory can see but not smell, because rational adult humans, despite their brains and their memories, occasionally hallucinate and dream (and feel, painfully, experiences they may never in fact have had).

The embryo's simultaneously reproductive, developing, and thinking existence, therefore, to Preyer, resembles, but is not identical to, hallucination or dreaming. And as such, it is (tweaking Preyer's terminology a bit) a hauntingly powerful variation on something that looks and smells a lot like environmental memory. The driving force, the mist, the smog that keeps embryos always quasi asleep (and with stuffy noses) may not be narrative memory, it may not be working memory—they are not sleeping in order to re-live their self-indulgent self-narratives. But (and like bacteria or algorithms), the thought and sensitivity that whistle up embryonic fear and sleep still, nonetheless, constitute a type of irrational, diffuse remembering. Preyer's insistence that his readers bracket the brain in their understanding of embryonic development, in short, opens the door to an inrush of uniquely embryonic memory—laced even, perhaps, with a faint, limbic whiff of nostalgia.

A question one might ask is where these dreamy embryos, fading away in the positivist laboratories of the nineteenth century leave the coalescing and dispersing dust motes, animalcules, and molecules that coated the surfaces and interiors of Buffon's reproductive milieu. If there is still here the collision of life and thought that transforms the nonhuman assemblage into a biopolitical assemblage, and if there is still the sensitivity and memory things less lost than never had, where is the environmental shift from material space to material time? Where are the *topoi* slicked over and replicated as, themselves, affect and memory—the reproductive atmosphere as archive, data hoard, or storage shed?

One non-answer to this question—in multiple parts—is that by the end of the nineteenth century and beginning of the twentieth, most commentators had moved away from the theory of "aura seminalis" that both Buffon and Hément had ignited and wafted out into the air, in favor of more apparently materialist definitions of reproduction. What remained, though, was the debris. Even as the model of the world as a ball of swirling reproductive particles disintegrated, the waste that it left behind—and the waste that kept, despite its despised character, throwing up awkward affect and sensitivity—refused to leave the stage. Minot, for example, while explicitly rejecting the "notion of the 'aura seminalis,'" and writing that "fecundation implied a material contact of the semen with the ova,"[70] also defined "sexuality" as "a *relation*[71] of substances or forces," and "male or female sexuality" as "an intracellular relation of parts, some modification of the interplay of forces within the cells."[72] So far, so good—no embarrassing, extraneous, dirty matter leaving a rotting, decomposing odor to bother (or not) dreaming embryos.

Tripping over such positivist precision, however, an intellectual successor to Minot, Şakir, lands himself in an altogether more grimy environment. Şakir's stated goal in his work on embryonic development, growth, death, and decomposition is, as a medical doctor, to advise lawyers who might be called upon to try cases of abortion or infanticide in a new, post-revolutionary Constitutional Ottoman Empire. His first exhibit as he presents his expertise to his audience, however, is Preyer's pinned down anencephalic infant or fetus, and how this sort of specimen transforms any conversation between law and medicine into an exercise in absurdity. His next is to play up the dispersed, environmental, atmospheric activity of life and reproduction. And his third is to cite, explicitly, wasted, decomposing embryonic material as the repository of political life, thought, and memory.

Although, he writes, neither the physicians associated with the law nor lawyers themselves, would consider "children" (*atfal*) born without a head to be living—and although specialists of embryonic development can speak with certainty on such matters to judges—scientists can never be sure that some sign of viable life has not escaped notice. Might it therefore be worthwhile, he continues, to explore the viability of a newborn child born with a brain "filled with water, soft like paste or dough, and embellished or traced with lines like tangled grass?" Şakir's answer is given in the question: undoubtedly such an investigation is worthwhile; no matter how carefully an autopsy (that is, an abstract narrative) might be conducted, observers can never know that evidence (in its infinite particularity) of life does not exist—and that such a child might in fact live or be alive.[73]

By criticizing both what he sees as the narrow definition of "life" accepted by a conventional legal establishment and the brain as the seat of both thought and life, Şakir is capturing, incongruously, a ricocheting Preyer. Both use the anencephalic fetus as a stepping stone to an argument about the unbounded qualities of both thought and life. More to the point, though—borrowing Preyer's pins—Şakir also questions the validity of these definitions by, specifically, enchanting his audience with a description of an apparently useless, putrefying brain in a "child" that might, nonetheless, be, or have been, alive that rivals, in poetic intensity, the reanimated pregnant woman laid out on Demangeon's table. Associating the brain with liquid, with unformed or unfinished dough, with filigree, and with tangled grass, Şakir hints that the life and thought of this unraveled embryonic material are physically embedded in flourishing, artistic, or vegetative accumulations. There is a faint, cold breath here of Buffon's brain-like womb whose conception of ideas and life of its own by no means detracted from its (positive) "vegetable" quality. There is also, given Şakir's later career, a chillier and stronger breeze heading straight in Martin Heidegger's direction.[74]

For now, though, it is mostly worth emphasizing that Şakir does not simply remind his readers and listeners, as Preyer does, that the anencephalic brain is absent. Rather, he takes a damp step further—describing this brain as a different kind of matter. Şakir's anencephalic brain is connected but diffuse, fluid like water, capable of growth like dough, and networked or open-ended like filigree or tangled grass. The description of the dead brain that by no means suggests a dead or unthinking "child" is deliberately beautiful—and Şakir's departure from Minot's (not to mention the Young Turks') positivist embrace of rationality as the basis of political belonging leads him to the same theory of embryonic life and thought that the far more spiritually inclined, humanist, Preyer, had reached thirty years before. The lawyers are incorrect; there is a politics of life prowling around in the tangled grass of flourishing reproductive matter that neglects, spectacularly, to reach a unified endpoint. And this biopolitics resonates because it similarly neglects to disentangle the sensitivity and vitality of this growing, dispersing, living fluid.

When Şakir turns to the waste and refuse that leak out of the biopolitical system he is implicitly embracing, the text becomes even more creepily
poetic and evocatively disturbing. He writes at length—and with much
salacious detail—about his personal knowledge of the evidence physicians and lawyers might skim off of the bodies of decomposing fetuses
and newborns turned into trash. He includes in his study, for example, an
extended chapter that addresses both the "incineration" of newborns and
their disposal in cesspools, toilets, and sewers, asking, as an opening gam-
bit, whether "burning or incinerating a child is a difficult and extended
task." In answering this question, he specifies with likewise much precision the steps a perpetrator must take—noting in particular that burning
will last as long as the "dried and desiccated corpse" has "soundness and
energy." Practically, therefore, even a very small corpse must be treated
for longer than a half an hour, especially without chemicals, and the oven
must never be opened because an open door can both compromise the
task and produce "bad smells." If the incineration is undertaken properly,
though, it is an easy task, and even a "servant girl" who may have given
birth "secretly" can do it.[75]

Şakir's discussion of disposing of newborns in sewers, toilets, or cesspools is less hypothetical—based, he avows, on specimens to which he had
access. He writes, for example, that he once examined a male newborn
child, of around one kilo and 250 grams, that had been immersed in the
bottom of a sewer; the cranial bones were scattered, but showed no signs
of crushing or refraction, the body was decomposing, the tracheal artery
seemed healthy, the head and heart were filled, although the condition of
the blood in the heart made it clear that the immersion could not have
been an accident; the stomach and liver contained air and were rotten, the
intestines were occupied by a thick, filthy material, and many of the body
parts were similar to yeast; the child, Şakir concludes, had likely been in
the sewer for around a month.[76]

Fascinated in these accounts by the transformation of coherent, potentially cognitive or psychological life and thought into incoherent, irrational, thinking sensing assemblages, spread out over environments, Şakir
also delights in the translation, in turn, of this accumulated, assembled

matter and information into filthy, yet still shrill and vocal, trash (just a quick bit of trivia: Heidegger was exactly 20, further north, when Şakir presented these lectures). Şakir's writing is, in short—and forgive the bare, un-ironic exegesis—horrific. It also, however, peels away better than most the protective, misleading, and scaly coverings that can obscure the, sometimes also horrific—even if effective—nostalgia of classic (nonhuman) biopolitical life. Şakir's understanding of the role of the medical expert in relation to trashed reproductive material and information leads inexorably, tugging at that flayed skin, to a reevaluation of all environments as reproducing, decomposing, and remembering—physically, vitally, affectively, on top of one another.

Şakir himself, in fact, eventually mocks his self-appointed challenge as a medical expert—namely to determine whether the disposal of reproductive material is valid or not, and thus whether a crime has been committed. Yes, he writes, physicians can try to determine whether the fetus, stillborn, or infant was or was not "trash"—whether it was viable or unviable before it was destroyed. But—as important as it may be to make a determination of "trash" or "not trash" for the purposes of trials—doing so is next to impossible. It is also beside the point. Given the evidence, all evidence, both everything *and* nothing in the reproductive realm is, and is not, trash. Both everything and nothing is reproducing and—via reproduction—everything and nothing is thinking, achingly, about experiences that can never, and should never, be narrated. When Şakir describes the disposal of reproductive material—be it a decomposing newborn in a sewer or the filigree-like absent brain matter of the anencephalic fetus—he thus, compulsively, backs away from any overt mention of inert "waste." Even when he conjures up, swirling, the fire, water, and sewage into which the simultaneously reproducing and reproductive embryonic matter gets itself digested, he reconfigures what he conjured into a variation on, essentially, storage systems.

What concerns him in his analysis of incineration, for example? It is not whether or how the infant died, but whether and how the fire might die—where there might be interlaced tangles and knots between the life or "energy" of the fire and the life or energy of the "corpse." The fire, Şakir

writes, now less poetically than pedantically, lasts as long as the corpse is
"sound" or "has energy," and thus even the dead body is translated into the
stored or potential energy it may or may not release into its environment,
or as part of an environment. Nothing, not even a "corpse," is ever finished
as a living, reproducing system. Nothing is ever wasted. And nothing ever
ceases to spit out, spark like, terrifying memories.

Or, switch methods, what concerns him in his analysis of the "child"
rotting in the cesspool? Not the "child"—although, true, Şakir does determine intent in this case via a reading of the corpse (the body was not in
the sewer "accidentally"). On the contrary, the purpose of taking stock
of each of the body parts or organs, and, painstakingly, carefully, obsessively, of how each of these body parts has changed, seems to be less to
search for the truth of life or death, and more to determine the nature or
quality of reproductive trash as a dynamic system. There was air in the
liver and stomach, filth in the intestines, and blood in the heart and brain.
This all tells Şakir that what happens in a sewer is not just decomposition or disintegration. It is also a process by which body parts begin to
resemble, copy, and replicate one another. Şakir is not simply celebrating
entropy or decay here—taking pleasure in the work of stored and potential
energy. No, the child's body in the sewer both copies itself and copies its
environment—as well as storing environmental information. It becomes
not just a variation on the reproductive biopolitical norm, but an archive
of nostalgic memory—*topoi* and *loci* saturated with information packing
an affective punch.

These ghosts are more serious than the ones that were flitting and tapping their way through the model room at the beginning of this chapter.
And they certainly unnerve more than the corridor of biographical trick
portraits that served as this case study's textual reservoir. Although they
are likely to pull you up short, though, keep in mind that these more sober
phantoms are part of the same family, subject to the same disintegration
into dust at the back of the box as their less—realistic seeming—tawdry
counterparts. The embryonic material that bubbles up in this chapter
and that, in doing so, plays up the nostalgia radiating out of the biopolitical collision of life and thought—this embryonic goo that transforms

environment and place not just into a complete, replete reproductive atmosphere but into a physical menagerie of memories and sensations—is a piercing case study because of both its life *and its afterlife*. It is key—from Buffon through to Şakir—because of how it lives, how it replicates, how it grows, how it thinks, how it feels, and how it decomposes, becomes debris.

The nostalgia of nonhuman political life is exhaled, in small, barely discernable wisps, when embryonic matter coalesces, grows, flourishes, reproduces, and thereby—as an assemblage—thinks. This same nostalgia, however, overwhelms all hint and tint of place, space, and ecology when the embryonic matter turns to waste. It is the difference between sensing a dim chill in the room, and the blinding, lightning flash transference of realizing that the room has moved suddenly backward to the moment when its hapless former inhabitant died, horribly. In short, a punchline to this chapter is that when nonhuman assemblages—in this case, embryonic atmospheres—reveal themselves to be a biopolitical model (or set of models, vanishing, again, into the distance, behind glass), and when these nonhuman assemblages also reveal, in turn, the inevitable collision of life and thought, the memory that they leave as debris across *topos* and *locus* is a memory tied up not just in their flourishing but also in their disintegration.

The mixed-up temporal materiality (nostalgia) of biopolitics—hitching a ride here with the now well-worn mixed-up spatial materiality of biopolitics[77]—is as comfortable in, and just as drawn to, waste, that is to say, as it is comfortable in and drawn to organized growth. Or, as Colebrook citing Deleuze has put it with reference to "eros beyond bounded bodies," "syntheses beyond the organism" do not presuppose a finite, tragic, death as end, but rather "intensities tending toward minimal thresholds . . . the movements of plants to the light, the movements of particles towards (and away) from each other."[78] In other words, the particles, regardless of whether they are coalescing (and reproducing) or repelling (and disintegrating), are still feeling, sensing, desiring, and thinking. More telling, they are becoming places and spaces that, because of their reproductive desire, are never quite securely fastened in time.

Or, to build a bridge—or a rickety footpath—from the slimy, biological case study inhabiting this chapter to the sere, informational, alphabetic case study peeking back from the coming pages, take some nails and pieces of wood from Jennifer Gabrys's work on digital trash. Gabrys challenges the conventional definition of rubbish as "a relationship between 'matter in place and matter displaced,'" by positing that "the very process of displacement can . . . give rise to places," and that dirt, therefore, has both more mobility and "'motility' or stickiness" than the traditional definition of trash suggests.[79] Debris, in short, makes places and also makes objects stick—despite the passage of time—to these fabricated places. Debris is, in this sense, nostalgia. Reproductive debris and (as) digital debris are only more so.

But there's an even stronger set of planks further on in Gabrys's book— fit for another, unexpected, bridge back, this time, to Chrostowska. Writing about the same troublesome digital archive that inspired Chrostowska, Gabrys likewise—from the direction of rubbish, trash, and waste—makes three key comments. First, she writes, nothing can ever exist, at least potentially, "outside the walls of the archive"; second, since an "archive can continually renew everything through digital operations," all "'waste' in the record can be rescued, instantly, as an item of relevance"; and third, therefore, "data is not lost because it is not archived . . . it is lost because it is archived, because it is digitized," inhaled into the "endless" particularity of the collection.[80] From this three-plank platform, Gabrys goes on to describe how the "electronic archive . . . of objects and data," via the "dual operation of disposal and recovery," thus raises the problem, especially, of "salvage,"[81] or, as she writes in a different part of the book, how contentless waste (like "spam and junk mail") can "acquire value through its circulation within particular spaces of value."[82] Her call, therefore, is for "a radical reconceptualization of waste itself."[83]

Gabrys's book is a brilliant response to this call—and in many ways the case study that unfolded over the past chapter has tried to echo this response. Nonetheless, you may still be wondering how it is that a story that started with shy ghosts, conjured into existence despite themselves, creeping into the model room late at night, just missing the departed musicians, has ended with a discourse on digital debris—and even that only after a protracted journey through a ghoulish embryonic wood teeming with headless, dreaming fetuses and reanimated screaming corpses, not to mention the spritely, lively molecules and animalcules flitting about in their generative atmospheres.

Here's how (a punchline): ghosts and digital debris bear more than a passing resemblance to one another, and not just in 1980s era speculative fiction.[84] Ghosts, like garbage (digital as well as reproductive), are dead things whose atmospheric presence provokes a start, a fright, a visceral response. Ghosts, like archives of unviewed data, like embryonic matter that fails, just barely, achingly, to meet, are—proverbially—nostalgic. This chapter, therefore, has ended with undead digital waste because it is, politically, the same thing as undead embryos and disintegrating reproductive material.

And so the main themes of this chapter remain: (a) there is a place in the history of biopolitics for unbounded accumulations of reproductive matter; (b) this place was marked off, charted out, dug up, excavated, and marked with a small, informational sign and a rope barrier over the course of two centuries of embryological writing; (c) given their style of reproduction—a dizzying coalescence of conceived thought and conceived matter, of perception and replication, of sensation and growth—these accumulations of reproductive matter may not just have a place in the history of biopolitics, they may also potentially be a biopolitical norm; (d) one synonym for this style of reproduction—for this transformation of environments into materialized space and materialized time, for the scattering of sensation and memory across *topoi*—is "nostalgia"; (e) nostalgia is the platform upon which biopolitics operates. And then there's the corollary that these stories reiterate with ghostly insistence: of all of the reproductive, flourishing translation of biopolitical places into biopolitical memories, the most efficient is that undertaken by trash. Debris reproduces; and its reproductive output is a repository of political memory, of nostalgia.

Alphabets

S ilted up in the debris left over from the party in the model room, hanging by bits of adhesive, briefly floating, then clattering down in the midst of the reverberating echoes of the departed musicians, are a number of placards—placards with names and affiliations; placards with explanations of the parts and bits of the fetal bodies on display; placards with menus, with dates, with schedules, with data. These placards, needless to say, or write, are repositories of alphabetic characters, of script, arranged, rearranged, and then disarranged as they fall to the ground in a suggestive heap, corners shredded and ripped off, centers saturated, soaked through, and then dissolved by some unidentified fluid on the floor. The second major case study supporting this book, then, concerns the biopolitical life and nostalgia of disarranged data (in letter form), the eradication of alphabets as an example of political life, thought, and memory.

Embryonic matter (the last case study) is an intuitive resort, vacation spot, for a study of nonhuman political life—even if it is less sunny and inviting for a study of nonhuman political thought. Data, generally, broadly, everywhere is also more than welcoming to such research— witness examples as diverse as anthropomorphic androids from late-twentieth-century television shows whose nonhuman credentials played out in an inability to handle grammatical contractions in English to the dynamic digital rubbish of Gabrys's tale. Less instinctive as a choice of case study in living, thinking information, however, is the stolid technology of script chiseled into stone, cloth, paper, vellum, wood, screen, and skin (or the backs of giant cockroaches). Nonetheless, hitching a ride with Baudrillard's immortally disgusted, forgotten gods on the automotive traffic that eats up roads in the same way that watches eat up time, are, here, collections of letters—the primordial data hoard—living, replicating, reproducing, remembering, and thinking, as nonhuman assemblages, even as they die, disperse, and transform themselves into trash.

Granted, in part this choice of second case study is an exercise in perversity. There is so much relevant material in the kingdom, dominion, and province of, say, surveillance, social networking, or the archiving of endless footage, material waiting to be mined and reconfigured into a story of data that lives, that reproduces, and that thinks, perhaps even as a democratic norm. Why not tackle this muscular, tentacled, flourishing, germane accumulation of experience rather than obstinately mucking about in the congealed dust of an obscure, precious (fussy-precious, not valuable-precious) historical moment meaningful to only three or four specialists too afraid to make the grand gesture? Two reasons. The first is that, although the Turkish Republican extermination of its earlier (Arabic) alphabet in favor of a new and improved (Latin) alphabet in the 1920s was more successful (scare quotes deliberately absent—give it its due) than many of its counterparts, it was also by no means unique.

Most of Central Asia, much of East and Southeast Asia, bits and pieces of South Asia, parts of all of the Americas, much of Eastern Europe, swathes of the African continent, Western and Central Europe[1]—presumably the message has been transmitted by now (everywhere and every place)—were hit with the fad to obliterate, replace, or simplify (the last defined in fascinatingly complex terms) the alphabets that happened to hold sway there. Killing alphabets in the late nineteenth and early twentieth centuries was an exercise in informational excess that rivaled the United States' National Security Agency's compulsive accumulation of chained up metadata in the early twenty-first century.[2] So although alphabets in cold storage may not be as obviously relevant to contemporary mass democracy and biopolitics as NSA agents on ice or embryonic material in the same frosty state, they are nonetheless vital, still zombie-like (or mummy-like—mourning the Rosetta stone), to any long-term history of the life, reproduction, thought, and memory of all sorts of accumulations of information and data.

The second reason for choosing alphabets over let's say the data that went into the Human Genome Project, now archaic, this time is (fairy tale style) that the difficulty of dealing with obscure, forgotten letters, alongside obscure forgotten gods riding around in cars that fail to go—the unpleasantness of taking the torturous trail through the thicket of sharp, decaying, pointed parts, rods, and spines of mechanical printing presses in order to prove the reproductive capacity of dead alphabets, and hence to observe their nostalgic political punch—is that the difficulty itself peels off and lays bare the life and thought of data in a way that easier trails, soft and nicely cushioned, do not. Images and arguments slide off of easy, slick surfaces. Suffer a bit, and they are burned in, branded there permanently, like, once again, writing on the back of a cockroach.

Or, try an analogy: destroying, painfully, a script, a system of writing eradicates narrative memory—a well (if paradoxically so) documented effect in scholarship on the subject;[3] it also, though, gives rise to a life in letters that scatters memory, affectively, across so many widely, wildly fluctuating systems, fields, and environments that it can never, ever, disappear completely. Choosing a case study unreasonably extraneous to contemporary biopolitical problems (the horror of the database with a life and consciousness of its own) similarly erases continuity in tales of posthuman politics. But its bad fit, its irritation, those same, or related, welts that it raises on that same, or related, skin, also force an annoyed, itchy glance at aspects of nonhuman life, thought, and nostalgia that scuttle off into hidden corners, no giant cockroaches, when the ordinary light—the day-time glare—of the model room is switched on.

Torturous thicket it is, then. Keep that image in mind while navigating the next few pages. Twisted, thorned vines twining around cracked firs broken in two by a strong wind that blew itself out a century earlier, lichen, bracken ferns, some toadstools by no means engaging or cute—each trying to suck the life out of the other before the first strangles it. Squash plants don't like forests, but they aren't alone in their fecund ferocity. Examine, therefore, first, a series of exterminated alphabets, stalled cars, and malfunctioning algorithms—all smashed precariously together into a tottering accumulation of data and metal, their similarities screeching in close, whining, slow proximity. Then consider a more lucid arrangement. The alphabets, cars, and algorithms, set side by side, despite the earlier collision, nonetheless all live, reproduce, move, and replicate in the same way. They also all remember, nostalgically in, across, through, and saturating nearly identical milieus—reports from language councils, advice on ameliorating traffic, and high colonial scholarship on the necessity of simplifying non-European languages and alphabets. And then end, finally, with a glade, with the point—pointed end of a marker, sticking into the wet ground marking the way out—that the dead alphabet, as a case study in the biopolitical life of unbounded data, is, like embryonic matter, a living, reproducing, thinking assemblage whose politics resides in its wanton, unrepentant nostalgia. Dead alphabets, remembering, repeatedly, forever, are also alive, flourishing, reproducing, and democratic.

In the name of false hope and dishonest clarity, though, let's start this case study with a deceptively straightforward, or initially, only slightly curved, history of the event. November 1, 1928: a clean, new Turkish Republican parliament, fresh from two decades of total war, unanimously passed Turkey's "Alphabet Law."[4] Arabic script, the script of six hundred years of Ottoman Turkish literature and governance, now hovered between the private and the criminal—officially, Turkish letters were (and always had been, by the magic of official memory) Latin, and public and private correspondence in Arabic letters, after June 1930, would be illegal.[5] The Alphabet Revolution, so called, spiraled out, fractal-like, and twisting

up, revolving and winding into seemingly countless other, similar script
rotations and spins, hacking, buzz-saw like, into Cyrillic and Chinese as
well as Arabic, especially in Turkic-speaking countries that had dug up,
in the backs of disused bookcases, new leases on revolutionary life. But it
also remains a stable and stationary flag, pillar, and craggy monument (all
mixed up together), a unique moment, in mainstream Turkish Republic
political memory—immediately and shockingly effective, narrated nowadays in the form of a sort of doubtful waking dream in which all traces of
Arabic characters disappeared one night in 1928, to be replaced, the next
morning, by their Latin counterparts.[6]

Remembered as such, the Alphabet Revolution has been a touchstone
for evaluating the success of other reforms—or, perhaps more accurate,
it has been a huge, immovable boulder used to pin down or smother the
more skitterish revolutionary efforts that failed to live up to their potential. Here's a fun one: in 1967, at a conference on Turkey's automotive
traffic problems, one of the participants, Hüseyin Sarıkardeşoğlu, advocated removing irregular vehicles from Turkish streets—in particular, the
shared semi-private taxi vans, or *dolmuş*es (literally "stuffed"), that operate in most of Turkey's cities—in the same spirit in which Arabic characters had been eliminated from Turkish script.[7] *Dolmuş*es, Sarıkardeşoğlu
insisted, could be destroyed and replaced with a coherent, regular vehicu-
lar system just as Arabic writing had been destroyed and replaced with a
coherent, regular alphabetic system.[8]

Sarıkardeşoğlu will, fear not, receive much rehabilitative praise as we
hack our way through the thicket of this chapter (or try, skitterish in a
different way, to pick a path across its chaotic urban street). Before these
rehabilitative gestures, though, one must admit that Sarıkardeşoğlu was
swept away a bit by his own rhetoric (it happens); his comparison, therefore, did not strike the popular chord of practical common sense toward
which he was aiming his small wooden hammer. Nor did his reference
to the Alphabet Revolution impress most of the other participants at the
conference, all of whom chose not to revisit it. And yet, even if the note
rang false, listen to it reverberating for a moment alongside other faint
suggestions—a thin, barely noticeable line (senses switched again) keyed

into the finish of a newly painted car—that, oddly, collections of letters and collections of vehicles have more in common than one might think.

The lead story on the first day that the newspaper, *Milliyet*, went to press in Latin rather than Arabic script, for example, had to do with regulating the flow of traffic and taxis, alongside the price of cars generally, in the new Turkish Republic.[9] Yes, it's the sort of coincidence of which false memories and false analyses are made—too simple. But it is evocative. But turn, nonetheless, regretfully away from it to something better grounded, back, perhaps, to Boym, who writes that technology and nostalgia do relate to one another in one way (even though computational assemblages cannot feel the ache of irony) in that each is "about mediation."[10] And by mediation Boym means—invoking the fact that nostalgia has always been "connected to passages, transits and means of communication"— everything from the "invention of writing in ancient Egypt" to "railroads" to "the modern metropolis" to "the timetables" regulating each, upon which nostalgia is always gamboling and "playing [its] tricks."[11] Check the footnote—each of these aspects of nostalgia trips after the other in the space of a single paragraph on a single page. There is something strangely, nostalgically, tangled up, that is to say, in the jumbled heap of writing systems, transportation systems, urban systems and the tricky, tripped up timetables that fail to link them all together. Traffic, alphabets, and time have an eerie affinity.

Sarıkardeşoğlu, then, was on to something when he pushed his proposal, even if it wasn't cold, resilient revolutionary necessity. The link, if tinselly, that he forged (or twined) between the revolution of alphabets and the revolution of *dolmuşes* sends up, as the two hasps make contact, a slight, sparked spurt of memory, of political thought, and of political life. It posits that the political value of letters, of graphic characters, rests (or, in fact, fails altogether to rest) in non-linguistic, non-communicative, repetitive, rotating, and mechanical operation, rather than in their remarkable ability to record or represent subjective or psychological cognition or encounter. Revolving alphabets, as revolving *dolmuşes*—shifts in script as shifts in stuffed buses—shunt hysterical narrative to the side (centrifugal force) while, humming and whirring along, they weave together an alternative lack of story, replete with memories. Taken together, alphabets—like transportation systems—are thus best expressed as extended, mechanical systems, especially when in the midst of revolution.

Moreover, and especially given Boym's tricks with timetables, alphabets, and automotive traffic, as weirdly similar systems, hint that both memory and classic, clichéd, kitschy political memory are more operational or mechanical than they are subjective or psychological, more spread out across failed urban structures than simmering in the hot brains of cool political agitators. If we take Sarıkardeşoğlu's argument as a starting point, in other words, the political memory of the alphabet as well as the political memory recorded within the alphabet is technological, environmental, and living. It is not subjective, and it is certainly not subject-forming. It is a freakishly effective variation on, as embryos were as well, nonhuman nostalgia. Letters as traffic lead to memory as a borderless collection of affective, particular, disordered objects and signs.

But before pursuing this line of argument, an embarrassing (it will be quick) mention of intention is in order to press this initial dense coalescence of script and cars into something with enough gravitational pull to keep this chapter revolving: when Sarıkardeşoğlu insisted that the *dolmuş* posed the same problem to the Turkish nation state in the 1960s that Arabic script had posed in the 1920s, he was not making a point (unaware, as he was, of the problem with pins plaguing this study) about how writing or memory work. His antipathy toward the *dolmuş* instead reflected a more general fear of what the *dolmuş* did to (and said about) Turkish streets and Turkish civilization. *Dolmuş*es, like Arabic characters, were disorganized, unnecessary, and uneconomic. More so, and also like Arabic characters, they could be replaced with one bold blow. They could be eliminated as a system in a single effort of will and then supplanted with a more efficient system. Dump the particular bits and pieces into the scrap heap and exterminate the vexing unified narrative. Solving the "*dolmuş* problem" quickly might be difficult, Sarıkardeşoğlu argued, but the "*dolmuş* revolution," like the Alphabet revolution, had to be quick. Immediate and total action was the only acceptable course: *dolmuş*es would be destroyed in another Republican revolution, replaced with a network of larger vehicles, while *dolmuş* drivers were introduced into this newly created environment.[12]

More intention (it's almost finished—we'll be back among the dissolving, non-subjective assemblages soon): Sarıkardeşoğlu's enthusiastic vocabulary of revolution and reorganization, however, once again, did not meet with much approval during the conference at which he floated it. He was older than most of the other participants present, and his metaphor reflected a moment in Turkish Republican history that had for the most part passed by 1967. Nonetheless, even though most of the conference goers cautioned against eradicating the *dolmuş* system altogether—noting, for example, that doing so would deprive not only the *dolmuş* drivers of their livelihood but also many Turkish citizens of their mobility—they also agreed with Sarıkardeşoğlu's assessment of the "*dolmuş* problem." The *dolmuş* system created a breach in traffic flow, it was disorganized, it stood in the way of a rational bus service, and the constant stopping and starting of *dolmuş*es on the street created horrible traffic jams.[13]

A year after the conference on Turkey's tied up traffic, De Leuw-Cather, an American company charged with conducting a feasibility study for the construction of the first Bosphorus Bridge elaborated on the theme of the erratic, destructive *dolmuş*. The *dolmuş* system, the report stated, employed a pointless (or, infinitely pointed) "circular pattern," and in this way threatened the rational automotive infrastructure that would culminate with the bridge.[14] The experts writing for the company recommended, therefore, that "that *dolmuş* and minibuses be restricted from operating on the Bosphorus Bridge, and that express bus service be the only means of public transportation allowed."[15] At the same time, however, they also noted that confining the *dolmuş* system to "the arterial street system" would compound existing problems there.[16] The assumption on which De Leuw-Cather preferred to operate, in the end, calmly, with none of Sarıkardeşoğlu's enthusiasm, was that sometime in the future, *dolmuş*es would be eliminated altogether. Like Arabic characters, *dolmuş*es were on their way out because—and, once again, like Arabic characters—*dolmuş*es did not suit a modern, streamlined, rational transportation-communication structure.

The intentionality is now safely back in its box. Ponder for a moment longer, though, the divergent fates of Arabic script and disorganized *dolmuş*es. The *dolmuş* system, after all, is still alive and well throughout Turkey, whereas—with a few exceptions[17]—Arabic script has disappeared. There are a number of straightforward explanations for these different outcomes. The Turkish political climate in 1967, for example, was differ-. ent from the Turkish political climate in 1928, balmy, less prone to freak purges. And, indeed, it is entirely likely that had the *dolmuş* system existed, and had it existed as a civilizational problem, for Mustafa Kemal Atatürk in the 1920s, *dolmuş*es, too, would have been eliminated. There is no reason to assume that some intrinsic quality of the *dolmuş* system saved it, whereas some intrinsic quality of Arabic script left the alphabet vulnerable. It could very well be that, by 1967, social engineering of the sort that would destroy the mobility of a large portion of Turkey's population was unattractive in a way that social engineering of the sort that would destroy the literacy of a large portion of this same population, in 1928, was not.

But where does this conclusion leave Sarıkardeşoğlu? Do we really have to ignore or silence him—write him off as a dinosaur or a nostalgic crank? Is it not possible to take Sarıkardeşoğlu seriously—and to remain open to the possibility that the *dolmuş* system and the Arabic alphabet have been similarly threatening to Turkish nationhood? If they are similarly threatening, and yet each experienced such different treatment at the hands of the Turkish Republic, then there is a hint at least, of some other interpretation of their differing revolutionary fates. Perhaps, after all, mobility is and has been more important to Turkish citizenship than literate memory is and has been. Perhaps destroying and replacing the means by which citizens move about a city has been unthinkable in Republican Turkey in a way that destroying and replacing the means by which citizens record and remember their past has not.

These conclusions, though, are no more satisfying than the easy references to the vague move to a gentler mid-century political climate. It is difficult to believe that the *dolmuş* system survived whereas the Arabic alphabet did not because mobility trumps memory in Republican Turkish politics. As much as commentators have described the Alphabet Revolution as a deliberate attempt to create a clean slate[18]—in fact to alter the Turkish population's memory of an Ottoman past[19]—it is hard to accept that similarly altering the urban landscape, eradicating the *dolmuş* system, was off limits to Republican social reformers. If Republican revolutionaries did seek to destroy historical memory as they eliminated Arabic script, why not destroy urban irregularities in the same way and for the same reason? Why would letters and memory be vulnerable to demolition in a way that mobility was not? Why are *dolmuş*es still snarled up on Turkish streets whereas the Arabic alphabet is safely ensconced in "heritage" sites?

One way around this problem is to reconceive both writing and memory—and to trot out, once more, the potential usefulness of nonhuman nostalgia as a framing device. Suppose, for example, first—with Sarıkardeşoğlu—that the force of alphabetic systems, like the force of traffic systems, is physical and material rather than symbolic or linguistic. Suppose that dysfunctional alphabetic systems like dysfunctional traffic systems pose problems not to cognition or communication, but to flow or circulation—that improper alphabets are irrational because they, like *dolmuş*es, are erratic and not streamlined. And, just to maintain momentum, suppose finally that properly political memory is nonhuman and nostalgic, an operation within or throughout mechanical or symbolic systems rather than a linguistic narrative of a past event.

Clothing ourselves in these suppositions—and hopefully, now, after 50,000 words, they are more than just suppositions—the preservation of the *dolmuş* system and the eradication of Arabic script lend themselves to more satisfying, warmer, cozier sets of interpretations. Most comforting, they hint that the removal of Arabic script from the Turkish landscape was, itself, a memory operation, alphabetic trash transformed into something resembling nostalgia. As a corollary, although less comfortable and more provoking, they also suggest that the destruction of alphabets, in Turkey and elsewhere, nowadays one of the easy targets—such clumsy, tactless, wanton modernity, they should have known better—becomes evidence of the value of memory in these Republics, writ large, rather than evidence of its disposability. Trashing the alphabet—the thing that is supposed to help us remember—in aid of better memory (the claims of the various reformers), in fact, can be taken seriously. When scripts and traffic are one, and when the nonhuman potential of nostalgic recollection peeks out from behind or under the traffic cones, these reforms are no longer the acts of malicious or incompetent modernizing monsters.

Here, then is the first twist of the path through the bristled thicket navigated: there is a faded, hazy confluence of cars and letters—of traffic patterns and alphabetic patterns revolving, spinning, and then lifting off, eradicated—hovering at the edge of the horizon. Trashed alphabets and dead or snarled traffic systems, overlapping and underlying one another, together, posit a different type of political memory, an extended, physical, embedded, operative memory that has nothing to do with narrative and everything to do with operation. They play up the potential of environmental memory with a physical punch—and pointless, circular, having no use for communicative bridges, automotive, linguistic, musical or otherwise, they insist, centrifugally, on the nostalgia that seeps into the debris and garbage silted up on the side of the road and the margin of the page. The nonhuman nostalgia of letters in flux, in other words, is, if not established, at least intimated, insinuated into the warm initial argument that protects one from the thorns in the thicket. Next, therefore, comes the second confluence—dead alphabets and glitched data or badly programmed algorithms. When the letters are both mechanical and informational, their nostalgic quality hitches itself, unerringly, to their reproductive potential, and to their life as well.

That the new Turkish alphabet, with its Latin characters, is more computational than Ottoman Turkish, with its Arabic characters, has appeared intuitive to many commentators. Geoffrey Lewis, for instance, whose account of the language reform does not attempt any explicitly computational analysis, nonetheless begins his discussion of the alphabet revolution with the following:

> Turkish writers on *dil devrimi* (language reform) do not usually deal with the change of alphabet, which for them is a separate topic, *harf devrimi* (letter reform). A brief account of it is given here for the sake of completeness, since the two reforms are obviously linked, arising

as they did from the same frame of mind. The purpose of the change of alphabet was to break Turkey's ties with the Islamic east and to facilitate communication domestically as well as with the Western world. One may imagine the difficulty of applying the Morse Code to telegraphing in Ottoman.[20]

A few pages later, Lewis continues, quoting Nicholas Negroponte, director of the Massachusetts Institute of Technology's Media Laboratory in the mid-1990s, that "at the word level, Turkish [written in Latin script] is a dream come true for a computer speech synthesizer."[21] An interesting, if subtly so, progression of propositions. Follow closely. First, Lewis states that Turkish historians of the early Republic have treated symbols (letters) and narrative (language) separately. Second, he continues, the shift to Latin script weakened religious belief ("ties with the Islamic east") while facilitating telegraphic code. And third, he states that Turkish written in Latin script suits nonhuman speech synthesis. In a single paragraph—think Boym with her Egyptian writing, railways, technology, and timetables— Lewis stakes out, with stable markers, no crumbling monuments here, a field of play for the nonhuman nostalgia of digitally inflected letters-as-data. New Turkish written in Latin characters is fundamentally computational. Its history is embedded in the history of computation and code, separated from subjectivity and narrative, and its greatest ally—desultorily dreaming of it and feeling it—is the computer speech synthesizer.

There is, however, also more going on in this computational history of the Turkish alphabet revolution divorced from human concerns and wed to dreaming machines. Yes, historians of the alphabet revolution have set up a divide between symbolic characters (the alphabet) and communication (language)—and have thereby hinted that alphabetic execution supersedes alphabetic message transmission. And yes, these historians have been tempted to invoke code, computation, and computational synthesis in their discussions. Telegraphing in Ottoman was hard work. In addition, however, this story of a shift in alphabets as also a shift in computational data, of writing symbols as digital processing is a tale of less cold and pure computational nostalgia in the early Turkish Republic. It is a portrait of memory, via writing, that is necessarily computational, nonhuman, and packing a physical thump.

But where did this memory, this nostalgia that was burgeoning, flooding, out of wrecked, discarded characters, replicating computationally across algorithmic systems, glut and torrent next? The schoolbook story of the moment, at least, is clear: after the overnight cleansing, with buckets, mops, and lye, of all traces of Arabic script, Atatürk, benevolent leader and teacher, toured Anatolia with a blackboard, educating bureaucrats and villagers alike about the value of coherent, well behaved script systems.[22] Soon, especially as Latin script facilitated widespread literacy in Turkey, so the story goes, no one mourned the lost Ottoman language—or, if they did, they were quiet about it. Hale Yılmaz has demonstrated that this popular story of the Alphabet Revolution is more nostalgic than accurate. In fact, she writes, the change in Turkish script occurred gradually and sometimes haphazardly—while both the act of Parliament that brought new written Turkish into being and the implementation of this act reflected a complicated social and political reality.[23] But this reintegration of reality into the tale only reinvigorates its nostalgic force.

According to the November 1928 Alphabet Law, for example—and here the collection of discarded, yet still quivering trashed letters start to do their work—different types of Arabic script would have different life spans as the revolution went into effect. By the beginning of December 1928, all advertisements, subtitles, signs, and newspapers would switch from Arabic to Latin characters; by the beginning of January 1929, all books, and government, bureaucratic, or other institutional communications would use the new letters; and by the beginning of June 1929, members of the public would have to use Latin characters in their transactions with government or private institutions.[24] "June 1930," Yılmaz writes, was "the absolute deadline for all public and private transactions, including all printed matter such as laws and circulars to be in the new letters."[25]

This gradual transition from Arabic to Latin script makes social sense—don't forget the policy hindsight and the rational intentions that go with it (they live on as stubbornly as disorganized writing systems). If the change had been as sudden as nostalgic narratives have suggested it was, the revolution would likely have collapsed and crashed. It is reasonable, as Yılmaz implies, that Turkish social engineers would have tried to make their policies palatable to an albeit punch drunk population. But this step-by-step transition toward Latin script also plays up a different sort of life, a different sort of thought, and an altogether, radically different type of memory than the schoolbook story. It quietly hints, for example, that Turkish alphabets—whether Arabic or Latin—were already, had always been, like all letters, everywhere, like all hoards of data, strip mined and collected without thought of collation, part of a computational, nonhuman, yet biopolitical logic, valuable for their operational rather than for their expressive qualities, resonant because of how they moved, revolved, replicated, and, themselves, remembered.

Go back to the law (just this once—you were forbearing about the intentionality before). The timetable—already ripped, tricky, and tripped up—of scripts to switch, and in what order, is telling (and riddling). The first set of scripts—the most influential, apparently—that would shift from Arabic to Latin were advertisements, subtitles, signs, and newspapers, each strings of letters that act, repeat, and reproduce rather than communicate. Advertisements, subtitles, and signs, especially, are, and often by definition (an equally operational verbal endeavor), sets of letters that do things rather than mean things (and yes, I am insisting here on a dichotomy). As a classic example of the active letter string, the street sign, for example, thinks through traffic patterns—it makes traffic operate, function, or fall apart. There is a reason, indeed, that Baudrillard seats immortal automobiles feasting on roadways alongside immortal gods feasting on nothing but time in his incomprehensible bourgeois dining room. The alphabetic symbol on the street, the sign, has almost nothing to do with expression or communication, and almost everything to do with being, itself, part of a material, environmental system or extended, symbolic, machine.

But advertisements and subtitles, too, operate, scatter debris across landscapes, and therefore, themselves, live and remember. It is the job of subtitles to shift symbols—they "translate," and thus carry, letters and words back and forth, from one meaningless context to another, rather than producing or communicating messages or meaning. They carry, on creaking backs, collections of particular letters from one place, dropping some along the way, perhaps, and then deposit them in another place, in the process always evoking an earlier experience that their readers and listeners, ignoring them, in any case, at the back of a dark theater, never had. Advertisements, likewise, as operational, informational, computational sets of graphic symbols littering landscapes with their notoriously dripping, polluting affect almost need no further explanation in this scenario. If letters do deign to be seen in advertisements, it is not to communicate, it is—in Pruchnic and Lacey's rhetorical, computational sense—to move, to reproduce, to act as information acts in computational contexts. Like street signs and subtitles, they are both digital and reproductive—and as they reproduce, they saturate landscapes with political memory that is not only memorable, but nostalgic.

So even before the Alphabet Revolution concerned itself with private or public correspondence (which would, belatedly, straggling and forgotten, change its form only a year and a half after the promulgation of the Alphabet Law), and even before it concerned itself with bureaucratic transactions or political or economic exchange, it tackled the letters that meant nothing even as they worked and reproduced across everything. Script that operated, that replicated, that did its own thinking, that worked as a machine in symbols was script ready for revolution. Script that replicated, reproduced, lived, and remembered, polluting and transforming environments as it did so was politically vital. Script that communicated— contrarily—was an afterthought. It is true that communicative writing eventually entered the revolutionary battlefield as well. But its expressive character disqualified it from participation in the initial revolutionary enthusiasm. Revolutionary letters, like revolutionary traffic, and like replicating embryos were the centerpiece of the tricksy timetable of shifting script that Parliament published—and published in the name of charting out a proper, modern, biopolitical democracy. Staid, communicative letters—those that tell stories and express subject positions—could come along for the ride, but they were largely irrelevant.

The newspapers and magazines that were supposed to shift at the same time as their billboarded counterparts, I should note, have sneakily evaded this part of the story—hiding, somewhere, under a thicket. In part, they've hidden because their role in the tale is more complicated than that taken by subtitles and street signs. Newspapers, in fact, were initially a notable failure in the revolutionary spectacle—utterly unsuccessful as they made the case for the new alphabet. "Readership dropped sharply," Yılmaz writes, for example, "when they began printing completely in the new alphabet."[26] "Some newspapers and magazines," she continues, even "shut down due to the ensuing financial crisis."[27] But failing to circulate, dying, and decomposing in a field of decaying digital letters does not disqualify these sheets and papers from their revolutionary function, nor does it undercut the capacity of their nostalgic, reproductive life in a modern biopolitical state.

If newspapers' value is determined by their capacity to circulate, after all—to do the same thing that traffic does—then newspapers too, dead or alive, are always active, replicating, and reproducing, are always part of the same living, digital mechanical-symbolic infrastructure that street signs are. If newspapers die because they fail to move or cycle rather than because they fail to communicate, then newspapers are no different from *dolmuş*es or anencephalic fetal matter. The letters in fact process better, reproduce and remember with greater vigor, as the meaning beads up and sloughs off of them, dripping into the parched field of meaningless revolutionary ideology. They are certainly more computational when stalled in their endless circles than they are when carefully read and digested by the thoughtful new citizens of a new republic. Circulating or stalled, that is to say, alphabets in newspapers live and think in the same way that any other processing symbol does—not from the message that they transmit, but because of the work they do, and because of how they replicate.

Second twist of the thicket, then, now navigated: collections of letters, dead, trashed, and revolving, are identical to both traffic and to digital information. Alphabetic systems in flux, traffic systems snarled, and algorithmic systems glitched can sit at the same table, together with the bored gods, remembering—and living.[28] Now, though, the question becomes whether the particular, affective memory of this alphabetic garbage, the experiences and feelings scattered across digital and physical fields, forests, and systems, is linked specifically—look again at the embryos—to reproduction and reproductive waste. Are alphabets really biopolitical life, and are their memory operations really something like the reproduction of classically living things? Loaded questions—and so on to the next bit of the thicket.

Given that nobody involved in script reform—Turkish or otherwise—has a good idea of what, precisely, in a revolutionary context, letters are supposed to do (they certainly aren't supposed to do anything so prosaic as representing ideas or psychological states), "live, reproduce, think, and feel the glorious repetitive tapping of nostalgic recollection" seems as good an answer as any. And, given the phonetic logic permeating these alphabetic revolutions, this may actually also be one of the better answers. Once phonetic logic becomes the grease that eases the alphabetic revolutionary turn, living, thinking, reproducing, and repeatedly tapping the root of affective non-experience become, in fact, a necessary bit of labor of letters on the move.

A general, and obsessively familiar, problem plaguing all nineteenth- and twentieth-century script reformers, for example—at least those with phonetic pretensions—was the paradox of trying to represent with a finite collection of particular signs (or objects), the infinite variations on sound that a human voice, as an abstract unity, could produce. Oddly (perhaps—choose your politics) here, the problem of the particular in this paradox thus adhered to the symbols (the letters) while the problem of the abstract inhered in the supposedly material voice. Less oddly, the nonhuman side of this non-equation was the collection of horizontal, and particular things (again, the letters), while the human side of the non-equation was the unity of the single, narrative voice. The implicit solution to these frustrations, therefore, suggested a problem less of arithmetic (x letter = y sound) than calculus (or, obviously set theory, and in turn Chrostowska's and Baudrillard's nostalgia): the set of particular symbols necessarily trended toward (a closed, small, bounded, algorithmic, or computational) infinity, the limit, as ever more matches to minutely varied sounds were presented to a waiting public. The symbols had an unfortunate tendency, in other words, to keep replicating and reproducing among themselves, in their cozy, closed set, with the exterior limit never reached.

Turkish linguists were adamant, nonetheless, that the only rational, revolutionary letter was a letter that existed in an ever elusive one-to-one correspondence with a single sound produced by a Turk communicating in Turkish (so much for rational numbers). And a proper, revolutionary alphabet, in turn, therefore had the simple, straightforward (as in a line, never segmented, stretching on forever) task of aiding, phonetically, vocalized human interaction.[29] Republican revolutionaries wanted letters to act as symbolic markers of what they believed to be a more real or material human linguistic process. A simple process.

And so, as a result, the logic of reform that they developed rivaled in irrational, complex, infinite, Mobius strip-like recursions and expansion the most freeform fractal generating program still plugging away on some fourteen year old's salvaged 1990s era desktop. Keep the limit point in mind (if never, obviously, in sight—vanishing as it does, parallel to the embryos, in the dark recesses of the model room) here: in order for a set of letters to participate in the revolution in the name of phonetics that Turkish (and other) social and political engineers introduced to them, the phonetic quality of these letters *could not yet exist.* In the revolutionary present, there could be no representational or expressive letters—only letters that would move or work in the name of a future phonetic rationality, in the direction of the limit point. Combining phonetic with revolutionary logic, in other words, transformed letters into narrowly computational or algorithmic strings of repetitive, reproductive, embedded information, forever processing—and never, as Buffon's animalcules and dynamic reproductive clouds of attractions likewise never were, at rest.

Linguists outside of Turkey grappled in even greater frustration with the horrifyingly fecund alphabetic symbols that proliferated wildly out of what was supposed to be cool, clear, streamlined obsolescence, death, and coherence. And these linguists also, in turn, ran up, repeatedly, against the iterative qualities of the scrapped, trashed script, still banging ferociously against the lid of the coffin—processing, with abandon, toward infinity and zero. The linguist C. R. Lepsius, for example—an influential forerunner to the Turkish linguists who facilitated the Alphabet Revolution[30]— devoted much of his writing to the inappropriate, gratuitous generative and reproductive capacities of the letter systems he was trying to tame. His own proposed Standard Alphabet was already immense—dismissed by his contemporaries as too unwieldy for practical application.[31] But his peers had no idea what Lepsius was battling, what reproductive monsters of late-twentieth-century sci-fi fiction and film had trotted back to contaminate his mid-nineteenth-century certainties; his defense of phonetic simplicity, which remained central to the logic of not just the Turkish alphabet reform, but to shifts in alphabets in other states as well,[32] framed, inexorably, a scene of reproductive mayhem, in which life, death, thought, reproduction, and memory collapsed, blissfully, into one another, mocking any attempt to keep the door of the space ship (never mind the coffin) sealed and closed.

Lepsius, however, is nonetheless still usually read as an advocate of letters that are simple, that do representational work, and that are part of finite—if large—sets. Letters in his texts are inert signs, and nothing more than signs. They are derivatives of spoken human language.[33] He is also, though, if you watch closely what he allows the signs to get up to when one's back is turned, an advocate of letters as data that live—of alphabetic systems that are an early, primordial variation on the database with the freakish, reproductive sci-fi consciousness. Lepsius develops at length, for example, his claim that his proposed alphabet would "bring the orthography hitherto used in science into more exact conformity with the laws of physiology, and to adapt it to practical purposes."[34] From there, he insists that the fact that all existing alphabets—even "the two great alphabetical systems of Asia"—can be "contained" within his own alphabet both "justifies" and "demands" an attempt to bring these results to pass.[35] Moreover, he concludes, bringing the Standard Alphabet to fruition in places where no existing alphabet exists is even more urgent: "the sounds once being known," Lepsius states with malicious simplicity, "the signs are easily applied."[36]

And so, at best, at its most staidly dynamic, this story Lepsius tells is still, already, a story of, here, finite, functional alphabetic algorithms at work. In the first situation, Lepsius argues that the mere potential for an all-encompassing set of symbols to replace existing "Asian" symbols demands an initiation of this process of reproduction and substitution. Phonetic logic and phonetic rationality require that symbols shift, appear, disappear, and realign. In the second situation, the existence of an empty alphabetic set, the vacuum, likewise cries out for repletion, for the computational process that might begin generating symbols to populate, carefully, rationally, the set. Although the first is more complicated than the second, each process is finite, functional, and indeed computational. Neither seems to hint at the grotesquely fecund space station, now nothing more than a bursting, splitting container of reproductive madness, hurtling, silently, nostalgically, through empty space.

Wait a moment, though. After presenting these and similar examples of the potential work of his Standard Alphabet, Lepsius sets in motion a different data-driven process. In addition to these functional algorithms with their specific endpoints or goals, Lepsius hints at the existence of alphabets more in line with Leuckart's (or Lovecraft's)[37] world, alphabets derived from and exulting in replicating shifts that can continue processing infinitely—and alphabets that, therefore, dysfunctionally, begin to think and remember and feel and sense on their own. First, for example, Lepsius notes that even his own docile, well-trained alphabet can, itself, grow and shrink, simplify or enlarge, depending on the work that it is doing.[38] His alphabet, in other words, is not just a set of symbols. It is also a set of reproductive and computational processes—it changes when its input changes. As such, his alphabet presents the possibility, at least, of other, less functional, more feral, disheveled, and uncultivated alphabets that might not only change with changing input, but trend toward pathology with this changing input.

The relationship among consonants, vowels, and symbols, for instance, is a relationship in particular that can, according Lepsius—as well as those influenced by his work—tip an alphabetic system into, precisely, a glitch,[39] a computational error, or a fecund, thorny thicket, growing always bigger and higher, out of some sadistic fairy story. The apparent simplicity of the one sound-one symbol rule, in other words, can trigger a dangerous situation in which an alphabet in the midst of digital shifting or reproductive reinvigoration can have a distinctively computational as well as oddly embryonic accident—an accident in which alphabetic symbols cease to have any correspondence at all to human speech sounds, and instead work, think, reproduce, and remember on their boundless, environmental own.

Entering into the nineteenth-century debate over the consonantal versus syllabic character of the ancient Hebrew alphabet, for example, Lepsius flags—with this flag almost immediately sucked, disappearing without a trace, rather than slowly sinking, into the fluid mire, the tip gone before his back has even turned—this potential problem. Arguing that later interpretations of the Hebrew alphabet as consonantal—that is, absent symbols for vowels—were incorrect, Lepsius states, first, that a "consonantal alphabet would presuppose by far too abstract a phonic doctrine on the part of its inventors," and second, that "intelligible" writing requires that there be "written signs for the principal and most expressive vowels."[40] Lepsius concludes that the early Hebrew alphabet must have started as a syllabic alphabet—with signs for both consonants and vowels—and only later started taking on consonantal qualities.[41]

Lepsius's attempt to restore the purity or "intelligibility" of a decayed or decadent ancient Asian system classifies him, complete with a sharp, cleanly typed label, hanging from a pin, as a nineteenth-century European scholar of problematic civilizational difference. That path is well trodden; give it a wave, but turn in another direction. As soon as you've turned, you'll run head on into a different sort of stench and decay. This stink, though, derived as it may be from unexamined (don't lift the lid) imperial assumptions, is a stink reminiscent—in a variety of ways, in a number of nuanced, slimy tones—of Şakir's likewise less than humane, civilizationally questionable, decomposing fetal matter. It is a decay, like filigree, like nostalgic, tangled grassy heaths (the tip of Darwin's head just visible over the horizon), in that it is anything but inert. This decayed system in fact is, in death, far more dynamic than it might be in a caricatured life and health. Regardless of whether he characterizes the presumed change in the Hebrew alphabet as decay or not, after all, Lepsius still writes—as Şakir does, of dead embryonic matter—under the assumption that alphabets are not static. They are shifting, changing, thinking, and reproducing even if this change is gradual and geological, rather than intellectual or biological.

Second, and voicing the despair of the nostalgic keeper of unviewed archives and misunderstood furniture, Lepsius's primary criticism of the consonantal alphabet is that such alphabets are "too abstract." The symbols in such an alphabet are dissociated from specific instances of human speech (the classic phonetic problem of the alphabet inverted and reasserted here). And, as a result, these letters inhabiting consonantal alphabets are secretly, exasperatingly prone to doing other, non-phonic work—threatening always, therefore, to dwindle, as a set of particular objects, even as human speech sounds proliferate in their infinite variety.[42] The one-to-one correspondence between human sound and symbol that characterizes the functional alphabetic process in Lepsius's universe is replaced in this example of a dysfunctional alphabet by an inverse relationship between sound and symbol. As sounds are made, symbols trend toward zero—a death almost as horrifying, subjectively if not computationally, as reproductive infinity.

Moreover, and unsurprisingly, this problem that Lepsius attributes to the glacially eroding, decaying, disintegrating Hebrew alphabet is also the problem that—according to Turkish observers as well as Turkish Revolutionaries—plagued Turkish written in Arabic script: Turkish, a language supposedly poor in consonants but rich in vowels was misrepresented, for centuries, by Arabic, an alphabet poor in vowels but rich in consonants.[43] Such an apparent mismatching of sounds and symbols created a situation in which—in the words of these nineteenth-century commentators—Ottoman spelling became a matter of "whim"—while printing, which required manipulating "more than 480 typographic characters," encountered huge technical and financial obstructions.[44]

Or, as Frances Trix has put it in a comparison of the Albanian and Turkish alphabet reforms, the "multiple equivalencies" between sound and letter that typified Turkish written in Arabic script "constituted a main criticism of the Ottoman Turkish alphabet."[45] While challenging the idea that phonetic simplicity was the sole engine driving alphabet reform,[46] Trix points out that "a single letter could represent multiple phonemes" in the Ottoman writing system while, at the same time, "multiple letters could stand for a single phoneme."[47] The problem with Turkish written in Arabic script—according to nineteenth- and early-twentieth-century commentators—then, was that, with digital or algorithmic abandon, it left the "equals" sign with nothing to do.[48] There was no equality in such an alphabetic system, and there was little representation. Instead the letters acted on their own, moving restlessly, endlessly toward some unspecified, future reproductive lack of a goal. Whether they were obliterating orthography by capriciously moving all over the place, or forcing typesetting machines to grind to a halt—proliferating beyond any reasonable mechanical bounds—these letters operated as a data hoard that put the most insectoid reproductive aliens and the most poignant of falsely remembering computers of the mid-twentieth century to shame.

They really got to work, however, not when they were enjoying their apparent phonetic irrationality, but when the revolutionaries started to try to fix the problem and, spinning, pin the willful script in place. Turkish written in Arabic letters may have demonstrated the digital threat of alphabetic characters, as data, proliferating out of control; but it was the shift in script itself that gave these letters a platform, a field, a forest, a dining room in which to repeat and replicate, with gratuitous abandon, and with prosperous, thriving nostalgia. Or, more bluntly: Turkish written in Arabic script was not the problem. Yes, old Ottoman Turkish, rather than new Republican Turkish made more apparent the likelihood that letters could and would act, think, and replicate on their own, detached from phonic rationality or relevance. But the real moment of reproductive, nostalgic biopolitics occurred in the switch from Arabic to Latin script.

What had been a problem of mismatched sets became a problem of infinite iteration. The process of shifting from a multivalent system to a system that—at some limit point—would create pure, singular equality gave the alphabet, as a thinking system, free rein. And in the way of these processes, within the gap between the smooth, never punctured, abstract narrative and the collection of particular, dissociated objects, a nostalgic world or environment in which symbols could meditate and replicate, detached from human linguistic sounds tumbled into existence. The process itself made possible an environment in which symbols could and did remember and secrete their memories. The Alphabet Revolution itself allowed strings of letters to act, symbolically, as matter, machine, and information all the way to zero—or to infinity if it was more satisfying.[49]

This conclusion, though, immediately leads to yet another quick new twist in the trail through the thicket: what—ideally in detail, in particulars possibly never experienced, but nonetheless pressing—did the nostalgic memories of the infinite sets of written letters produce or preserve? A number of commentators and scholars have addressed this question and begun to sketch, in fuzzy charcoal or fading watercolor, the contours of what seems to be a distinctly alphabetic mode of remembering—even as many of the contemporary commentators, those wrapped up in the revolution, tried to contain the informational, chemical explosion ignited by alphabet reform. Lepsius, for example, insists that since the "basis" of all alphabets is "the physiology of the human voice," and since "the human voice has its natural bounds, beyond which no development of sounds is possible," alphabets, even as they shift, must necessarily be contained: "the apparent infinitude of articulate sounds does not consist in a boundless extent, but rather in an endless divisibility, within assignable limits." For Lepsius, then, if infinite alphabetic iterations occur within a set rather than beyond set boundaries, these iterations are both comprehensible and controllable. They are a manageable infinity.[50]

The logic underlying at least one precursor to Republican Turkey's alphabet revolution—the so-called "military writing" that the Young Turk government promoted prior to the First World War—was similar to this logic that Lepsius kept letting off of the leash, bounding and defecating all over his well-maintained European field of inquiry. Following the Ottoman Constitutional Revolution of 1908, the Young Turk government established a committee (Şakir was doing other things) to look into reforming the existing Ottoman Turkish alphabet. This committee proposed the de-linking or separation of Ottoman Turkish (that is, Arabic) characters,[51] primarily in order to save printers the difficulty of "deal[ing] with three or four forms for each letter."[52] In 1913, Enver Pasha, the Ottoman Minister of War, instituted this form of writing within the War Ministry, first for telegraphing, and later for all "official correspondence within the ministry."[53] Once again, therefore, alphabets here become a

mode of both transport and computation. Telegraphy becomes the cata-
lyst that changes them, and the assumption underlying this change is that
the recurrent separation or division of letters could be controlled in a way
that the recurrent extension or expansion of letters could not.

But how and why would reformers as diverse as Lepsius and Enver
Pasha hit on this seemingly obscure point—this idea that if internal division replaced external expansion, the problem of alphabetic infinity might
be solved? Why would division within a set be desirable to these disparate
figures in a way that expansion beyond bounds was not? What sort of
memory seeps out of these givens? One possible response to these questions is that when figures such as Lepsius and Enver Pasha emphasize the
ostensible manageability of infinity within an alphabetic set—and the
unmanageability of infinite alphabetic expansion—they are making a case
for letters that are productive, or reproductive, even when these letters
are not necessarily comprehensible.[54] They are positing that the potential
infinitude of divided letters, like thinly sliced segments of embryos, within
a set, can do something that the non-productive, incomprehensible infinitude of letters, or any reproductive matter, beyond boundaries or borders
cannot.

And what these letters can do, it seems, is remember. As they proliferate
within the boundaries of a set, in fact, these letters create for themselves—
and incidentally, for humans as well—the familiar yet distinctive non-
space of nostalgic computational memory described as an ancient Greek
practice by Pruchnic and Lacey, as well as by Boym. They turn memory
into a set of processes—into the ongoing act of forgetting content while
shifting physical signs or symbols. As these letters iterate within their sets,
they demonstrate that political memory, at least in an alphabetic context,
is necessarily a variation on trauma or nostalgia—either the replacement
of the linguistic with the physical (trauma) or the replacement of the spatial with the discarded and materially temporal (nostalgia).[55]

Consider, for instance, the many types of political memory and nostalgia
that saturate stories of alphabet reform. First, there is national memory—
the trite historical memory of a collective bound by a fantasy of shared
culture. As many commentators on the Turkish alphabet revolution have

argued, a key goal of the Republican shift from Arabic to Latin script was in fact to re-engineer the Turkish version of this memory—to wipe out a collective Ottoman past in favor of a collective Republican present. Or, as Lepsius himself wrote from a different perspective, one reason that "foreign alphabets" had to be reformed, whereas "European alphabets" had to be left alone, is that collective European history demanded preservation whereas "foreign" history demanded reconfiguration:

> [given that] all European nations use one and the same order of letters as handed down to them by the Romans, who received it from the Greeks, who again received it thousands of years ago from the Phoenicians, they possess also the right of communicating the historical arrangement, as well as the characters themselves, to foreign nations.[56]

Once again, yes, this is some horrifyingly high imperial language. But, in checking off that box, you might also ponder, briefly, the reproductive, biopolitical, and computational (as well as imperial) implications of this passage. As much as Lepsius seems to be insisting on the unchanging quality of the "European alphabet," after all—and on the mutability of "foreign alphabets" (take the quotation marks as given from now on)—the stability of the former rests on a quite deliberate series of shifts. Indeed, the only difference between the European and foreign alphabets, at least as Lepsius describes them here, and at least as shiftiness is concerned, is that the European alphabet shifts over time, whereas the foreign alphabet shifts (or should shift) across nation or culture.

The inviolate collective memory that Lepsius seeks to preserve for Europeans, in other words, is as much indebted to ongoing alphabetic reconfiguration as the vulnerable collective memory of the foreigners he targets. In each case, collective memory becomes possible only as, first, written content or meaning is lost, second, alphabetic signs reorganize and reproduce themselves, and third this reproductive activity transforms time into a field of physical and material play. Losing the content of the written memory is thus a prerequisite, at least in Lepsius's universe, to producing any effective collective memory—"European" or "foreign." The set order (or series of orderings) of Lepsius's European letters indeed necessarily lose meaning as they shift from Phoenician to Greek to Latin to European languages. The patterns into which the letters fall may recur, it is true, but these patterns cease to express any specific content as they move in and out of language groups. Once more, though, this loss of meaning does not, according to Lepsius, presage the loss of Europe's collective memory. On the contrary, European memory—nostalgic, without any particular content, the content collected, horizontally, in archives no one visits—is preserved precisely as the letters order and reorder themselves throughout time and beyond meaning.

As a result, Lepsius's imperialism as well as Republican Turkish social engineering—not to mention the social engineering of the tasteless, embarrassing modernists in other states—take on unexpected connotations. If the Europeans with their "right of communicating . . . to foreign nations" both "the historical arrangement" and "the characters" of their alphabet seek, in doing so, also to export a set of norms, standards, ideas, concepts, or subjective relationships, for example, their project is doomed. Indeed, "communicating" any sort of message or meaning alongside a European-style alphabet becomes impossible. Non-representative, the letters are living, reproducing, content-free processes; they do and make things rather than expressing ideas. Collective memory inheres in their nostalgic reconfiguration absent any message, in their reproductive diversions across lively, living digital environments.

At the same time, however, if Lepsius's Europeans seek only to convey to his foreign nations this iterative process, the project becomes at best redundant. As Lepsius himself writes, "foreign alphabets" are *already* mutable. They are inherently subject to repetition and change. Just as "European alphabets" shift over time, "foreign alphabets" shift through something called culture. Neither Lepsius nor Turkish Republican social engineers, therefore, are even capable of the subjective or political violence that is so frequently attached to moments like the Alphabet Revolution. If alphabets operate as both traffic and information, if they reproduce like embryonic matter and in this eternal processing spew out clouds of nostalgia, then the collective memory of a population, imagined or not, is immune to damage—if not immune to contagion and pollution. Such collective memory certainly cannot be damaged via attacks, deliberate or not, on some static thing called an alphabet. Collective memory, on the contrary, is produced only as orderings of letters lose their content or message and begin, as boundless collections of living things, to reproduce themselves, to shift or reorder on their own. Destroying memory content is a precursor to producing collective memory. There is no content-based norm to export, impose, or for that matter, to subvert. Instead, there is nonhuman biopolitical life, which is held together in turn by nostalgia.

A second type of political memory frequently invoked in narratives of alphabet reform is literate memory. Not any less collective than national historical memory, this type of remembering is nonetheless most frequently associated with the modern citizen of the liberal nation-state, alone, reading a mass produced book or newspaper. As Yılmaz writes, "the expansion of literacy was a genuine goal of the proponents of alphabet reform," not least because Arabic script required "more than 400 pieces of type," whereas a "simpler alphabet would make printing more convenient and less expensive."[57] Caymaz and Szurek also point out, however, that modern literacy of this sort was an ethically ambivalent goal. Alphabet reform, they emphasize, does not simply involve replacing one system of signs with another; rather, institutions like the Turkish Language Council were transforming, through law, the formerly literate population of the state into the functionally illiterate—creating a type of "politically organized dyslexia."[58] When Atatürk introduced the new alphabet in gradually expanding concentric "circles," therefore—first to the literate elite in Istanbul, who were most likely to protest the change, and then to the urban and rural populations outside of Istanbul—he was fully aware of the paradox involved in promoting literacy through the enforced "dyslexia" of those who already could read.[59]

And, in fact, the Turkish Language Council itself had a complicated understanding of how these shifts in alphabets would reinvent both literacy and illiteracy. Doing everything it could to provide new spellings of all of the words that the population or "folk" currently used, the council also admitted that occasionally strings of letters would be neglected or "forgot-ten."[60] Moreover, the particular words or strings of letters that were least likely to make it into the new orthography were those that the Council deemed repetitive, irregular, or personal (such as inappropriate names).[61] Here too, then, the literacy promoted by the Alphabet Revolution would involve forgetting not only how to read but also the previous existence of what were now unspellable words. To be clear here: the Language Council was not banning and eliminating certain words *as* words (although it did that too); it was explicitly "forgetting" certain strings of letters as no longer spellable. The change was not at the level of culture or communication but at the level of alphabetic symbol as bit of data.

But was the enforced dyslexia of existing human readers of words really as relevant to literate memory as those who link it to alphabet reform sug-gest that it was? Or, for that matter, was an increase in literacy—in the number of people who could read or in the number of people with access to ostensibly more easily printed reading material—important to the pro-duction of literate memory? The computational qualities of the alphabet, and especially of alphabet reform, suggest that perhaps they were not. Perhaps a person actually reading, in other words—that ideal literate citizen—was a sideshow within the more vital interaction between revolu-tionary, reproductive alphabets, on the one hand, and literate, as opposed to national or collective, memory, to nostalgia, on the other.

Look, for example, at the challenges that both the old alphabet and the new alphabet apparently posed to literate memory: it was not the alpha-bets themselves or the words that these alphabets preserved that became memory, but rather the shifts both within and between alphabetic sym-bols that did so. More to the point (of the rusted out printing equipment, the thicket of metal spars no longer churning out paper and pages), if the complicated pieces of movable type associated with the old alphabet were an obstacle to literate memory because this system of type slowed or blocked the dissemination of written material, then literate memory was, once more, a function of the letters themselves rather than a func-tion of the reader accessing these letters. And if the solution to this prob-lem was to change the letters and thereby produce more and more written material, then, once again, memory resides in the ongoing, ever-present, repetitive iteration of symbols within a discrete set of boundaries, in the transformation, physically, of a landscape into a swampy, redolent mess of slime and information, rather than in the activity of the literate citizen, accessing this writing at some displaced future moment.

And finally—although from the opposite political perspective—if literate memory is also blocked by the widespread dyslexia that the new alphabet injected into the veins of an unsuspecting populace, then the issue at stake in alphabet reform is not that there will be fewer people around capable of reading texts in the old letters. It is not that the archive of texts in the old alphabet will be inaccessible and thus forgotten. It is that accessing the new letters will twist them into meaningless strings. It is that the "dyslexic" reading itself will, in the present, rather than in the future or the past, shift these letters away from content. It is that the archive of particular objects will, nostalgically, continuing reproducing, meaninglessly, materially, away from any potential unified, abstract, narrative. It is that the archive will become the bourgeois dining room set. Following the alphabet reform—just as before the alphabet reform—always, in other words, letters will move, reproduce, live, and remember on their own, eluding and evading the irrelevance of content-based human access.

In both situations, therefore, forgetting and remembering content become the same thing. Or, more precisely, content is forgotten so that literate memory can become a reproductive activity, nostalgia. Whatever content may exist either in the future streamlined printing process facilitated by the new alphabet or in the texts of the past archived and preserved in the old alphabet is less relevant to memory than the movement of letters in an ongoing, endless, repetitive, politically vital, and yet deeply satisfying present—in the dark, echoing, reverberating gap between the two. In the first scenario, literate memory is blocked by letters that, too complicated, cannot shift, repeat, or reproduce. And this memory is then released by simple letters that can endlessly shift, repeat, and reproduce. In the second scenario, literate memory is blocked by letters that should, to those previously comfortable with reading, have content, but, frustratingly, do not. And then this memory is released—if, according to Caymaz and Szurek, oppressively so—by letters that travel in concentric circles throughout the Turkish material environment, shifting, repeating, and reproducing. In each case, memory is not about preserving or transmitting meaning. It is about reconfiguring symbols as digital matter that lives and thrives—and that in the process secretes ever blossoming clouds of nostalgia.

And so the paradox of a Language Council that explicitly "forgets" certain strings of letters in order to promote literary memory becomes less of a paradox. Once again, writing here is not a means of preserving memory content externally so that a literate population can access it later on. And literacy has little to do with engineering more and more people able to read—able at, again, some potential future date to access a preserved memory, wrapped up in paper, taped smoothly, with no sticky, overhanging edges, to a well formulated, established experience. The Language Council was, on the contrary, completely unconvinced by the notion that if more people are able to read, then it is more likely that a memory, written down, will continue to exist. It imagined instead a far more dynamic relationship between literacy and memory that was immediate, ongoing, and material.

Yes, that is to say, memory is external in each of these examples of the nostalgia of reproductive letters, residing, with much uncomfortable wiggling, within strings of shifting symbols. But, as each of these examples also demonstrates, this externalized literate memory likewise demands the ongoing reconfiguration of reproductive letters, rather than a collection of pre-existing, inert characters that might convey meaning to be read later on. As Lepsius and Enver Pasha both made clear, the reason that infinitely dividing and repeating letters contained within a set are manageable is not because they are comprehensible; it is because they are reproductive—and evocative.

Sarıkardeşoğlu, then, with his strange inability to differentiate between stuffed minibuses snarling up traffic on the (potential) Bosphorus Bridge and disruptive, badly affixed, duct taped placards, covered in indecipherable, archaic alphabets, clattering to the ground or gumming up the works of humming printing presses, was not without some redeeming qualities. Alphabets, as hoards and stores of data, as the original hoards and stores of data, are not divorced, completely, from infrastructures (automotive or otherwise) as hoards and stores of machines. Letters, *dolmuşes*, and computational information (along with the algorithms that process them) have a family relationship, an embryonic genetic twist tie, affixing them to the same stake marking the end of the thicket. Each has a tendency, especially when in the midst of revolution, when the circular movement starts to get a little bit dizzying, to break down, die, decay, and dissolve in a remarkably political, and punchy, way. Each, given the tiniest chance, proliferates wildly, in particular abandon (or, once more, in the abandon of particularity), repeating and reiterating in the gap between the physical collection and the narrative intended to contain it. Each reproduces itself, and in the midst of this reproductive flourishing—remembers. Each lives—as Sarıkardeşoğlu hinted, unhappily—a biopolitical life central to democratic functioning, and the reproduction of each is a form not just of political thought, but of political memory, and of classic, if unbecoming nostalgia.

You ask, then, why, in a study relying so heavily, with perhaps overly optimistic trust, on just two case studies of organic and inorganic life, reproduction, and memory, the relatively meaty example of embryos in various states of study, presentation, and representation should be balanced by this austere—obscure—example of a moment of excessive nationalist social engineering in a little corner of not quite, never was, southeastern Europe. The reason—aside from the gratifyingly primordial quality of the alphabetic letter as bit of data (indecipherable rocks and papyrus crumbling into dust in the desert)—is that this moment showcases the unyielding normativity of the life of data and information in modern mass politics. The Alphabet Revolution is, in Turkey—as well as in other states that implemented or tried to implement similar shifts—a touchstone, a means of comparing and evaluating the effectiveness (leaving aside the ethics) of other moments of social engineering and citizenship formation. And yet, as the trek through the twisted, thorny thicket just laid bare, the story of this high point in republican modernity can easily be told without reference to any human citizens at all. The Alphabet Revolution works just as well as a story of alphabets—revolving.

Unlike the more obvious examples of the database that lives or information that becomes political, then, this tale of the death, decay, and then rampant reproduction of Ottoman Turkish script also shrieks out, in registers difficult to miss, like the sound of ancient, worn out brake pads on a snarled up street, that the life and thought of data collection is not just political, but a political norm. Alphabets in flux, like embryonic material spritzed into reproductive clouds and effluvia, live and reproduce; their reproductive activity is a variation on thought; this thought is, narrowly, memory—or nostalgia; and (and this is the bit where the alphabet comes into its own), the smashed up life, thought, and nostalgia of this information is both biopolitical and a biopolitical model. Citizens can learn something from thoughtful, spinning scripts. Alphabets, like embryos, are haunted, living things.

Conclusion

Look through the door of the model room and, as you're paying attention to the shapes and vague movements that you can only partially make out, in the dark, and as you're feeling the breath of a dim vanishing point, trip and tumble into the kitschy vortex of not quite properly remembered, oddly mismatched, peculiarly and irritatingly collated, yet always (uncomfortably) atmospheric, objects and affects of nostalgic experience. Nostalgic experience: this faintly embarrassing experience popularized by writers who have woken up from dreams both as long dead as the wuffling and galumphing mathematicians of the nineteenth century and as healthy and productive as the film trailers that recycle fairy tale villains into conflicted, misunderstood anti-heroes who are unfairly dogged by the overwhelming materiality—forests, ships, shoes, spells—that keeps remembering, vibrantly, all around them. This book, here, makes no claim for any more profound variation on that easy emotion. In fact, the only difference between this, here, and that, there, is that instead of the affect channeling through little girls shot in hazy sepia tones, the nostalgia here has seeped instead out of embryos and scattered, skittering, anachronistic alphabetic characters, bubbling over and staining with something evocative, but indecipherable, the digital pages of what is claiming to be a scholarly book. But, after all, perhaps this difference is not such an insignificant one.

After all, packing tightly together, in a crate lined with straw, just a little too small for the job, the 200,000 serial sections of the dusty embryo collection, the clear, neatly cleaned, cuboid glass and plastic cases that contain them, the fallen musical notes that plink to the ground when the musicians have left for the night, the stray bits of yarn, wool, and silk trailing from tapestries unraveled, rewound, and then hopelessly re-tangled, the placards full of pregnant letters digested, halfway, by mice and silverfish, now illegible, the ghosts—both the cartoonish ones that overturn half-drunk glasses of water, staining the tablecloths on Baudrillard's brand new antique furniture and the unnerving ones best not disturbed any more than necessary—the thickets with their faintly toxic, but never deadly, thorns along with the winding paths cut through them, a few forests, some cities silted up with debris and stinking trash, has been a deliberate, shameless exercise in provoking obvious, well-trodden nostalgic reactions (flattened, they are so well trodden). Being a scholar, you were likely unaffected by these feeble maneuvers (unless the creeping irritation of an argument not cleanly presented triggered the intellectual equivalent of a minor aggravation of the skin—a cognitive variation on drinking scalding hot chocolate just a tad too quickly, and blistering away the taste buds on the tip of the tongue; yes, that feeling).

If it makes a difference, though, there has been a purpose, if sometimes artfully hidden, burlesque style, to this shallow exploration of tired, even dubious (politically), themes—a purpose tied up, with twine, in the fact that this time, while wading through the shallows, we've left the little girls alone. We have focused, instead, on the waves, the water, the grains of sand, the rocks, the larval sea life, and the foamy whitish muck that sticks to the edges of the shore rather than being washed, properly, back into the sea. If the stuff is a better repository for nostalgic response than the people are—a conclusion, despite the sepia tones, shared by most commentators on the experience; little is more *dependent* on objects, on bits of disconnected information, and matter, even if displaced and badly understood, than the illness that is nostalgia—perhaps nostalgia, generally, is best described as an excretion of objects, bits of disconnected information, and matter, rather than of psychology and self-consciousness. Perhaps nostalgia is better described with reference to time materialized, irrelevant to psychology, than with time eluding capture (or cute, captured narratives of time elusive).

But this explanation or apology for the indulgent presentation of what should be dust-dry research has already inverted the logic driving (granted, while consulting a clumsily folded map, no GPS here) the rest of the book—it has pushed you head first back through the shards of the looking glass. The previous chapters, remember, did painstakingly hang up, drip drying, a step-by-step tableau of a thesis: step (1) biopolitical life takes as its norm unbounded, nonhuman life, the life of organic and inorganic assemblages; step (2) if nonhuman life is the biopolitical norm, then reproduction, that centerpiece of biopolitical engagement, is as much a nonhuman thought process as it is a process of bodily or genetic replication; step (3) more specifically, reproductive thought, as a variation on the thought of nonhuman assemblages broadly defined, transforms environments and atmospheres into spaces and locations of physically, molecularly embedded memories and sensory experiences; step (4) the thought proper to biopolitics (nonhuman politics in its most pristine form) is thus, by definition (extended definition—see chapter 3), nostalgia—and nonhuman nostalgia; step (5) modern political thought—if political thought is understood as a mass democratic activity—is, therefore, heaving ourselves over that last concrete stair, sprawling on the landing, the primordial nostalgia of (at least given these case studies) embryos and alphabets.

But the inverted version, drawn out blinking onto the stage now that you've reached the conclusion, is quicker: if nostalgia is the defining characteristic of reproducing objects and assemblages, and if reproducing objects and assemblages drive contemporary political engagement (pay no attention to the Žižek behind the curtain), then nostalgia is a key

component of contemporary political engagement. This conclusion is not
as trivial as it might appear to be. It is, for example, very much in keeping with various currents—out of the shallows now—in today's feminist
theory. And this study is, relentlessly—don't be fooled by the tangential
tone—a work of feminist theory, a study, in the classic mold, of the problem of reproduction (the reproduction of symbols as well as of matter)
in contemporary politics, a study of the centrality of life, bare life, the life
that keeps overwhelming the sterile spaceship, floating innocently in its
vacuum, and terrifying the cognitive, bad Cartesian, pilots (turns out he
had a brain all along), in modern mass democracy. It is a study that twists
into new, and hopefully pleasing forms, strands of conversations in the
intersecting fields of feminist engagement—conversations about the generative force of nonhuman assemblages and what political role this force
has and might play in democracies, about the affirmative potential of,
especially, data-driven biopolitics, and about the efficacy of embedded, yet
boundless, variations on thought and existence—of processing without
awareness, of memory without self-consciousness, of contemplation without cognition, and obviously of nostalgia without coherent narrative. It
takes seriously, again, despite the tone, the well-established feminist point
that purely human thought—a fantasy in any case—has become politically
anachronistic (if it ever had political relevance in the past).

So here we are, after the countless, repetitive, circular, and perhaps
badly strategized forays into forests, woods, and cities, still—dreamlike,
after opening the door at the end of the hallway that was supposed to
bring us home—returned to a well-marked, if not completely stable and
docile, field. An inhabitant, and a long-term inhabitant of the field, however, would posit that there are still a few more agricultural duties to
perform. First, a crop of some sort needs to be reaped—there must be
at least some gesture toward a reward for reconfiguring all of these piles
and heaps of theoretical soil (a euphemism—but a significant argument
thumping away throughout this book is that the non-euphemistic version
of this term is more valuable than even its sweetest smelling fashionable
alternative) into unexpected—and not always pleasing—arrangements.
There must be some purpose to banging on the pan and shouting about

nonhuman nostalgia until the ears ring and the glass cases shatter, shivering and splintering their sharp slivers to the ground.

In fact, there are two.

The first is in the style of, once again, classic feminist theory—it is that rearranging our terms in these ways helps, usefully, to reframe a series of ongoing political problems, and problems particularly relevant to feminist engagement, as—if not necessarily not problems—at least not the problems that everyone thought they were. Obvious, here, are the two case studies that propped up, tottering—three being a more architecturally stable, but less spectacularly circus-tent like, number—this book. Embryos and embryonic matter, or just reproductive stuff in general, have been terrifying classic liberal-democratic theorists and policymakers for centuries (or even millennia, if you want to define "liberal-democratic" broadly and incorrectly).[1]

More specifically, embryos, and human embryos especially, are a prickly, more than toxic thorn in the side, the edifice, the massive, elephantine hide, of political structures that take the embodied, rational, affective subject as a norm. This is because embryos, and human embryos especially, exist, as such, as subjects, only in the future (as potential) or the past (as part of the bodies that, in proper linear fashion, produced them). Embryos in the present are impossible to categorize—hence Louisiana's mesmerizing, absorbing, and ever-growing collection of microscopic, molecular orphans under guardianship—because they hint, coyly, at the dignity of the human without having anything close to identifiable human characteristics.[2] The ordinary liberal-democratic response to this paradox has been to open the ring to an, again centuries-old, blood spattered fight between those who want to privilege the future (potential human) quality of embryonic material and those who want to privilege the past (former body part) quality of this material. Embryos in the present are a nonstarter. More important for our purposes, neither of these positions, slogging it out on the parliamentary floor, has been all that helpful to feminist engagement broadly defined.

Rethinking thought, however, as the nostalgic byproduct of reproductive assemblages and environments, organic as well as inorganic—with embryonic matter a strategic example of such accumulations—attaches, with much adhesive, this mode of matter firmly to the present. The problem of what can achieve dignity as a potential human—that limit point never attained, even by the most well-composed, water- and air-tight, bounded, rational, embodied citizen, always a tiny rip in the skin, in the wall, in the hide—and what must welter away in the undignified realm of the part, Leuckart's misery, as we have seen, evaporates completely when the soil is heaped in a different way. Instead of trying to define elusive wholes and dizzying, dancing parts, democratic politics can (and historically, demonstrably, has) run instead on the dynamic, always present, thought of this growing, flourishing, reproducing matter—on the nonhuman nostalgia of reproduction in the here and now.

Exterminated and useless alphabets have posed a similarly ghoulish threat to political engagement in the democracies that have successfully (or even unsuccessfully) nailed them into a coffin and buried them. As much as the Turkish Alphabet Revolution is a touchstone by which other reformist efforts have been evaluated, for example, the specter (and this is not a metaphor) of Arabic script, of Turkish written in the wrong, Oriental, sylph-like, letters (cubic kufic and siyakat the stuff of papyrus and sheep registers), continues to haunt the Republic's public sphere. In part, the poltergeists have been summoned by those who claim to hate them most—a pre-fabricated model of counter-revolution, of protest-ideology, clicked, Lego-like into place once Arabic script became not only unofficial, but illegal. More so, though, the ghosts—the less mischievous ones—have menaced, seemingly, because of the memory that was or was not destroyed along with the old alphabet.

The blood spattered ring enclosing and restraining the proponents of the two, apparently dichotomous, responses to exterminated script, in other words, looks eerily similar—same swinging overhead lamp, same flickering bulb, and same rabid, baying audience—to the concrete floor across which advocates of variations on embryonic political status abuse each other. On the one side, there are those who insist that destroying the memories preserved, like the fragile, inherited pink glass tea set no one in the family knows what to do with, in the velvet lined box of the discarded alphabet was a sad and necessary part of modern state building. On the other side, there are those who retort that dumping these memories, shattering the tea set, splintering the box, was an act of vandalism, unjustified and indefensible by any political rhetoric. Each assumes that alphabets, snugly wrapping up memories, inhabit the not-now. Whether trashed and discarded or recycled and repainted, alphabetic characters are terrifying either because they take us backward, into a not-modern, not-progressive, not-civilized despotic past or because they take us forward, into a likewise not-modern, not-progressive, not-civilized authoritarian future. Like the response to the attack ostensibly undertaken by embryonic material, the response to their unwonted assault on the self-evident value of rational, embodied, affective, humane political engagement is to shove them into a sci-fi phone booth and push "go." Like embryos, scattered alphabetic characters fail entirely to take root in the now.

Also like embryonic material, though, the reconfiguration of normative political life and reproduction as the life and reproduction of nonhuman assemblages, and the reconfiguration of normative political thought as the primordial nostalgia that spurts, seeps, and wafts out of the reproductive activities of these assemblages—such assemblages, for the most part, not nearly as wedded to temporal linearity as their rational human counterparts have been—rearrange the ethical and political tokens in this game. The flickering bulb over the ring finally burns out, with a snap, and when the lights are repaired and turned back on again, the auditorium is empty. The antagonists, hurting each other over the proper protection of politically beneficial memory have a difficult time maintaining their aggressive, manic high when it turns out that the trashed alphabet—like trashed embryonic material—produces, creates, and excretes memory rather than letting it escape and scamper off into the woods through the fissures that formed when it fell to the ground.

Alphabets in flux, like embryonic material in clouds and polyps in crystals, are radically reproductive—and, as a result, they necessarily smear memory all over all the *topoi* and *loci* that they touch or contact. Given this shift, shimmering, in perspective—same scene with just a few crooked little imperfections to indicate the quantum alteration—alphabets, like embryos, can also exist, and have existed, comfortably, politically, bio-politically, and ethically in the present as well as in the past and future. Alphabets, like embryos, are the biopolitical and democratic now.

This first crop from the tilled field, then, is, once more, recognizable—related, in a family sort of way, to other products that have been flourish-ing in recent feminist theory. Things that have been taken, uncritically, as damaging to democratic engagement are, perhaps, not so. And indeed, this crop also resembles other produce that might be matured, using the same techniques, in the sifted soil spread out over this study (provided, always, that the aggressive squash plant doesn't overwhelm them). We've tended to the embryos and the alphabets. But other tendrils have also begun creeping up in the same set of beds.

Trash, garbage, and debris, for example, are by no means the demons of mass extinction, the harbingers of global destruction, or the swirling mael-stroms of human evil (swirls of something undoubtedly—but not neces-sarily narcissistic human self-criticism) in the middle of the Pacific Ocean that they frequently are in popular accounts of their monstrous flourish-ing and growth. A number of scholars—Gabrys most notably here—have already complicated the ethics and politics of rubbish in productive ways.[3] Implicit in the plastic bottle tops and candy wrappers occasionally spotted in the by no means pristine forest and thickets of these pages, therefore, is a complement to this pre-existing work: as reproductive political sys-tems, trash and garbage, too, secrete a democratically viable primordial nostalgia.

Or, consider more narrow subsets of this reproductive matter that has been served up, steaming, as case studies here, on the pink glass plates. One variation on embryonic material—the human clone—for example, is a celebrity of sorts in the realm of public policy: loud, relentlessly vis-ible, the disembodied repository of the fantasies and fixations of countless activists and observers. The human clone is, indeed, legally and liter-ally, as I said using exactly the same words in the Introduction, the very worst thing in the world—an enemy, in hysterical legal, policy, and ethics documents, of the human species, of "mankind," in a way that only two other evil figures, the pirate and the perpetrator of genocide, have been.[4]

Feminist theorists have already paused to wonder why the human clone should prompt such an extreme response on the part of policymakers.[5] Here, though, once more, a partial, additional rejoinder to this rhetoric begins to peek through. If the human clone is one, of many, variations on embryonic matter as a reproductive, nostalgic, and thus democratically engaged accumulation of matter and information, perhaps it needn't be tricked out in an eye patch and a wooden leg—or, full circle, stored in a less value-neutral version of the transparent, glass box (with air holes and Hannah Arendt in the audience), than those in the Blechschmidt collection. Perhaps an alternative political rhetoric of cloning, less terrified of the monstrous fecundity of the flourishing alien,[6] might start to form.

And then finally, one last additional example of where this path through the woods might take us, there is the data hoard. The alphabet, as a case study in living, reproducing, thinking, politically active computational information, once again, is a deliberately perverse illustration of the arguments meandering through these pages. It is indeed a database of sorts—but compared to, say, the NSA's data mining operations, it is what the Jacquard Loom is to corporate search engines or sci-fi artificial intelligence (nostalgic, in other words).[7] Taking on the problem of reproductive data from the perspective of the dead alphabet, however—initiating this shift from, if not an ethically inert perspective, at least the perspective of a relatively obscure and narrowly contained example—shoves us toward the reconfiguration of more lurid conversations about more ominous, pulsating problems in flourishing data, problems such as the NSA's surveillance policies.

If reproductive data, if the data hoard in general, is a political figure that engages, satisfied and replete, in nostalgic repetition rather than in the cynical use and manipulation of narrative memory, then perhaps data mining need not be defined as the newest totalitarian opponent, the surveillance activity most indicative these days of horrific, mass democratic sovereign states run mad. And, in turn, perhaps the data hoard is more appropriately a problem for feminist theorists—for scholars concerned with reproduction, thought, ethics, existence, and democracy—than it is a problem for the proliferating, like polyps or tribbles, rogue males who keep making breaks, variously, for Russia, Ecuador, and the virtual universe of TED talks. In short, that is to say, the first reward ripped from the converted soil of this study is that conversations about any number of democratic problems might redirect themselves into avenues at least less ethically, and ideally less politically, obvious or facile.

The second reason for dragging you through these thickets of sliced up embryos, not for the squeamish, and for demanding that you look at the musical notes shuddering, traumatized, on the floor of the model room, though, is more fundamental—and also perhaps more rewarding. It has to do with the fact that the trip through the forest, the examination, at length, of the reproductive material—in clouds as well as spread out on slabs— and of the sharp, pretty, useless script do, insistently, happen in the present rather than in the past or future. It has to do with the fact that the nostalgia excreted by these reproducing accumulations of data and matter can inhabit only an endless present—that the gap between the infinitely iterating collection of dissociated, horizontal particular objects and the infinitely smooth, opaque narrative that misses them is a temporal as well as a cognitive gap, a gap in which the repetition is satisfying because it maintains the sensory experience *as* experience, rather than giving it over to past or future story.

This style of thought and existence, this satisfied, repetitive, enjoyment of the present, is—especially now, in late liberal, never liberal capitalism— improper not just because it is (ostensibly) unproductive but also because it is implicitly immoral. There is too much joy in it. Nostalgia thus has not only a bad odor (and scratchy feel) to it, but an ethical whininess that sets it up against the educational, well-disciplined progress narratives already succumbing to cancer, to growth. Those objects, assemblages, and in fact people who trend toward the gap, the nostalgia—algorithms processing infinitely, accidentally toward Parisi's and Portanova's soft thought, archives of digital bits of stories never quite reaching saturation point and thus expanding, expanding, expanding, children appreciating a beetle, excessively, rather than participating in school time skits that reenact historic war crimes—are, variously, fixed, reprogramed, and cured. The repetition, the bliss of the present, the appreciation of the dust mote, isolated—each is politically improper.

If, though, political life and political thought do, and historically have, come together in, specifically, this sort of endless, disconnected, present existence, if reproduction—the biopolitical activity par excellence (Žižek out from the curtain)—is, itself, a variation on this radically embedded thought, if the primordial nostalgia of embryos and alphabets is indeed a democratic norm, then these cures, fixes, and patches are nothing more than a melancholy absence of remedy, a search for time that truly never did exist. It may be the case that this non-progressive, non-subjective, noncommunicative thought is open not just to toleration, therefore, but to installment as the most appropriate mode of political engagement. Or, alternatively, the dust mote is not just a supplement. Look at the 200,000 embryonic serial sections. But don't try to learn anything from them. Just look, smell, taste, hear, and feel.

INTRODUCTION

1. Nick Hopwood, "'Giving Body' to Embryos: Modeling, Mechanism, and the Microtome in Late Nineteenth-Century Anatomy," *Isis* 90, no. 3 (September 1999): 462–496, 492.
2. Jean Baudrillard, *The System of Objects*, trans. James Benedict (New York: Verso, 1996), 41.
3. Or, as Baudrillard continues, "an object no longer specified by its function is redefined by the subject, but in the passionate abstractness of possession all objects are equivalent. And just one object no longer suffices: the fulfillment of the project of possession always means a succession or even a complete series of objects. This is why owning absolutely any object is always so satisfying and so disappointing at the same time: a whole series lies behind any single object, and makes it into a source of anxiety. Things are not so different on the sexual plane. . . . Only a more or less complex organization of objects, each of which refers to all the others, can endow each with an abstractness such that the subject will be able to grasp it in that lived abstractness which is the experience of possession." Ibid., 92.
4. M. A. Hill, "Embryology," Blechschmidt Collection, https://embryology.med.unsw.edu.au/embryology/index.php/Blechschmidt_Collection.
5. Eric W. Boyle, ed., *National Museum of Health and Medicine: Guide to Collections* (Silver Spring, MD: Otis Historical Archives, 2014), 199–205.
6. M. A. Hill, "Embryology," Hubrecht Collection, https://embryology.med.unsw.edu.au/embryology/index.php/Hubrecht_Collection.
7. Ibid.
8. Susan L. Crockin, "The 'Embryo' Wars: At the Epicenter of Science, Law, Religion, and Politics," *Family Law Quarterly* 39, no. 3 (Fall 2005): 599–632, 610.
9. Defined as such, for example, in Janet Poole, *When the Future Disappears: The Modernist Imagination in Late Colonial Korea* (New York: Columbia University Press, 2014), 57.
10. As Jussi Parikka puts it, "the extension of life to inorganic processes follows from Deleuze and Guattari's philosophy. Life consists of dynamic patterns of variation

and stratification. Stratification is a living double articulation that shows how geology is much more dynamic than dead matter. This is obviously an allusion to ... Deleuze and Guattari's *A Thousand Plateaus*, in which the whole philosophical stakes of this enterprise are revealed. The intensities of the earth, the flows of its dynamic ... are locked into strata. This process of locking and capture ... organizes the molecular inorganic to 'molar aggregates.'" Jussi Parikka, *The Anthrobscene* (Minneapolis: University of Minnesota Press, 2014), 16.

11. Michel Foucault, *Society Must Be Defended*, trans. D. Macey (New York: Picador Press, 2003), 241.
12. Ibid., 241.
13. Famously or, at this point, notoriously, see Giorgio Agamben, *Homo Sacer: Sovereign Power and Bare Life*, trans. Daniel Heller-Roazen (Stanford, CA: Stanford University Press, 1995), 121–122.
14. Foucault, *Society Must Be Defended*, 243–244.
15. For a more extended discussion of the scholarly fate of "biopolitics" over the past three decades, see Ruth Miller, "Biopolitics," in *Oxford Handbook of Feminist Theory*, ed. Lisa Disch and Mary Hawkesworth (Oxford: Oxford University Press, 2015), 61–78.
16. For example, "'Life', far from being codified as the exclusive property or the unalienable right of one species, the human, over all others or of being sacralized as a pre-established given, is posited as process, interactive and open-ended. This vitalist approach to living matter displaces the boundary between the portion of life—both organic and discursive—that has traditionally been reserved for *Anthropos*, that is to say *bios*, and the wider scope of animal and non-human life, also known as *zoe*. *Zoe* as the dynamic, self-organizing structure of life itself stands for generative vitality. It is the transversal force that cuts across and reconnects previously segregated species, categories and domains. *Zoe*-centered egalitarianism is, for me, the core of the post-anthropocentric turn; it is a materialist, secular, grounded and unsentimental response to the opportunistic trans-species commodification of Life that is the logic of advanced capitalism. It is also an affirmative reaction of social and cultural theory to the great advances made by the other culture, that of the sciences." Rosi Braidotti, *The Posthuman* (Cambridge: Polity Press, 2013), 60.
17. See Claire Colebrook, *Death of the PostHuman: Essays on Extinction*, vol. 1 (Ann Arbor: Open Humanities Press/University of Michigan Press, 2014), 84 (parsing Brian Massumi) on the political force of the non-cognitive.
18. Agamben, *Homo Sacer*, 121.
19. In characterizing this trend in literature, Braidotti writes, "I am perturbed by this fixation on *Thanatos* that Nietzsche criticized over a century ago and which is still very present in critical debates today. It often produces a gloomy and pessimistic vision not only of power, but also of the technological developments that propel the regimes of bio-power. . . . This over-emphasis on the horizons of mortality and perishability is characteristic of the 'forensic turn' in contemporary social and cultural theory, haunted by the spectre of extinction and by the limitations of the project of western modernity. I find the over-emphasis on death as the basic term of reference inadequate to the vital politics of our era." Braidotti, *Posthuman*, 121.

20. Bruno Latour, *Politics of Nature: How to Bring the Sciences into Democracy*, trans. Catherine Porter (Cambridge, MA: Harvard University Press, 2004), *passim*.

21. Jane Bennett, *Vibrant Matter: A Political Ecology of Things* (Durham, NC: Duke University Press, 2010), 62–63, 95.

22. Or, obviously, when they do meet, in the form of global capitalism, the result is at best, a horror. Consider, for example, Cheah's interpretation of liberalism and bio-power in *Inhuman Conditions*, "I have merely attempted to locate the inhuman way of being human in the technologies of bio-power that enable the actualization of humanity through economic development. Instead of regarding the inhuman as an attribute, effect, or consequence of the global capitalist system *qua* product of alienation from our humanity, it would be more accurate to situate global capitalism as the terminal form of microphysical and biopolitical technologies, tactics, and strategies that stretch across labor-exporting and receiving nations. . . . What is at work here, however, is a form of inhuman production that cannot be regulated and transcended because it is the condition of possibility of humanity. It forms the concrete human being and all its capacities at the most material level. . . . This constitutive imbrication of human rights in bio-power does not inevitably lead to futility. Just as technologies of bio-power cannot be controlled for the pursuit of humane ends, they also exceed the terminal hegemonic forms (e.g., the state or the bourgeoisie) whose power rests on them. Since we have never known a human condition that has been purged of the inhuman, instead of seeing the inhuman as a fall from an ideal humanity, we should ask: How does the inhuman force field sustaining global capital induce effects of humanity and how are these effects contaminated?" Pheng Cheah, *Inhuman Conditions: On Cosmopolitanism and Human Rights* (Cambridge, MA: Harvard University Press, 2006), 231–232.

23. This is a deliberate overstatement. Much feminist theory has questioned this start divide. For example, "What if thinking were discordant with what has been taken to be life? To take thought and its capacity for separation seriously is at once simply Cartesian, but also demands a different thought of life: what is thinking life such that it can diverge from causal and efficient modes of reasoning? What is thinking such that it can ask the world-destroying question of Descartes' evil genius, the question of the non-being of this world? This divergence of faculties is generally attributed to Kant who separated the capacity to think beyond the given world from the capacity to know the world as given: if it is possible to think what cannot be known or given then even though this 'not knowing' places limits on theoretical knowledge it nevertheless opens up the possibility of acting as if something like pure Ideas were possible." Claire Colebrook, *Sex after Life: Essays on Extinction*, vol. 2 (Ann Arbor: Open Humanities Press/University of Michigan Press, 2014), 65.

24. Giorgio Agamben, *State of Exception*, trans. Kevin Attell (Chicago: University of Chicago Press, 2005), *passim*; Achille Mbembe, "Necropolitics," trans. Libby Meintjes, *Public Culture* 15, no. 1 (2003): 22, 30.

25. Agamben, *State of Exception*, 134–135.

26. As Latour writes in a mild critique of this trend, "that a human should speak in the name of several others is as great a mystery as the one in which a human speaks in such a way that he is no longer speaking at all; instead, the facts are speaking for

themselves through him. Someone who says 'I am the State,'—'France has decided . . .,'
is no easier to decipher than someone who knows what the earth's mass is, or can
quote Avogadro's number in an article." Latour, *Politics*, 70.

27. Wendy Brown, *Edgework: Critical Essays on Knowledge and Politics* (Princeton,
NJ: Princeton University Press, 2005), 86.

28. Marianne Constable, *Just Silences: The Limits and Possibilities of Modern Law*
(Princeton, NJ: Princeton University Press, 2005), 8.

29. "So I would pause at this point to make a minor conclusion. in terms of intellectual
history it is inaccurate to see a straightforward anti-Cartesianism in the very tradition that is often appealed to, today, to make the case for 'Descartes' error.' Even
Nietzsche—who would seem to be the philosopher to whom one might wish to
appeal in order to get beyond the Cartesian prison . . . was not so clear in attribut-
ing the blame to Descartes. Nietzsche even suggested that the modern assassina-
tion of the soul was actually counter-Cartesian and, for that very reason, utterly
pious. Nietzsche saw a religious fervor in modern philosophy's extirpation of the
soul, and a pseudo-Christian self-abnegation in the tradition, after Descartes, of
ridding the world and life of anything like the soul." Colebrook, *Sex after Life*, 2:60.

30. For one (of many) interpretations of the overlap of information and matter in this
realm, see "Yet the microchip, like the gene, requires, 'all the lateral-social articula-
tions and agentic relationships,' from . . . 'researchers' to 'machines' and 'financial
instruments,' in order to circulate in the world. Discussing these 'things' involves
being able to register the complex forces that bring them 'into material-semiotic
being.' This study does not advocate an approach that attempts to de-fetishize the
chip or electronics. Instead I seek to develop a method that can encompass the
apparent singularity of the chip together with the things it powers and the disparate
fields it affects." Jennifer Gabrys, *Digital Rubbish: A Natural History of Electronics*
(Ann Arbor: University of Michigan Press, 2011), 8.

31. Chapter 2 provides a more extended definition of "nostalgia," as well as literary history of the term, for the purposes of this study.

32. Pheng Cheah provides a useful definition of normativity (in relation, paradoxically,
to human rights) in his *Inhuman Conditions*: "Here, let me offer a schematic working definition of 'normativity' for a non-specialist readership. Simply put, normativity is that which confers the status of norm upon a maxim of action or a desired
state of affairs. It is the being normative of norms, that which makes a norm normative. Thus, normativity is that quality that makes us regard ourselves as obli-
gated to bring about a certain state of things or as being bound—etymologically,
obligation derives from *ligature*—by an imperative commanding or restraining a
certain course of action. Pheng Cheah, *Inhuman Conditions: On Cosmopolitanism
and Human Rights* (Cambridge, MA: Harvard University Press, 2006), 149.

33. "Frederic Jameson was correct to claim that Deleuzianism is today the predomi-
nant form of idealism: as did Deleuze, New Materialism relies on the implicit
equation: matter = life = stream of agential self-awareness—no wonder New
Materialism is often characterized as 'weak panpsychism' or 'terrestrial animism.'
When New Materialists oppose the reduction of matter to a passive mixture of
mechanical parts, they are, of course, asserting not an old-fashioned teleology

but an aleatory dynamic immanent to matter: 'emerging properties' arise out of unpredictable encounters between multiple kinds of actants (to use Bruno Latour's term), and the agency for any particular act is distributed across a variety of kinds of bodies." Slavoj Žižek, *Absolute Recoil: Towards a New Foundation of Dialectical Materialism* (New York: Verso, 2014), 6.

34. Especially to the extent that it upset, rather than reinforced, some of the more problematic human–animal interactions. As Braidotti writes, "the oedipal relationship between humans and animals is unequal and framed by the dominant human and structurally masculine habit of taking for granted free access to and the consumption of the bodies of others, animals included. As a mode of relation, it is therefore neurotic in that it is saturated with projections, taboos and fantasies. It is also a token of the human subject's sense of supreme ontological entitlement. Derrida referred to the power of the human species over animals in terms of 'carno-phallogocentrism' and criticized it as an example of epistemic and material violence. In their commentary, Berger and Segarra argue that Derrida's work on animality is not peripheral but quite central to his analysis of the limits of the Enlightenment project." Braidotti, *Posthuman*, 68.

35. And . . . it's out. See n. 33, Žižek, *Absolute Recoil*.

36. Thomas S. Kuhn, *The Structure of Scientific Revolutions* (Chicago: University of Chicago Press, [1962] 2012), 178.

37. Dragoş Chilea, "Le Régime juridique de l'identité génétique de la personne en droit européen," *Curentul Juridic* 43 (2010): 53–68, 55.

38. Emine Elif Vatanoğlu-Lutz, "Research on Embryos in Turkey with Ethical and Legal Aspects/Etik ve yasal açıdan Türkiye'de embryo üzerinde araştırmalar," *Journal of the Turkish-German Gynecological Association* 13 (2012): 191–195, 193.

39. Glenn Greenwald and Ewan MacAskill, "Boundless Informant: The NSA's Secret Tool to Track Global Surveillance Data," *Guardian*, June 11, 2013, http://www.the-guardian.com/world/2013/jun/08/nsa-boundless-informant-global-datamining.

40. A legal approach critiqued by Bertrand Pulman, "The Issues Involved in Cloning: Sociology and Bioethics," *Revue française de sociologie* 48 (2007): 129–156, 146, and a cultural approach critiqued by Sarah Franklin: "These pejorative associations with clones' sexuality" are linked to the idea of "a sexuality based on narcissistic identification (gay clones) and slavery [either as 'slavish imitation,' or in the association of clones with a worker class of slaves or drones]." Sarah Franklin, *Dolly Mixtures: The Remaking of Genealogy* (Durham, NC: Duke University Press, 2007), 27.

41. Helmut Illbruck, *Nostalgia: Origins and Ends of an Unenlightened Disease* (Evanston, IL: Northwestern University Press, 2012), 18–19. Svetlana Boym, *The Future of Nostalgia* (New York: Basic Books, 2001), xiii–xiv.

42. Reviewing the literature on this take, Boym, *The Future of Nostalgia*, xiii–xiv.

43. An approach to nostalgia critiqued in Alaister Bonnett, *The Geography of Nostalgia: Global and Local Perspectives on Modernity and Loss* (New York: Routledge, 2015), 101.

44. Alienating, as Bruno Latour notes, because "technology," unlike "science" is a little bit too close to the human world—hence "alien" in a horror-inducing monstrous

sense, rather than alienating in, say, a Marxist sense. As he writes in *Aramis, or The Love of Technology*: "As accustomed as we have become to the idea of a science that 'constructs,' 'fashions' or 'produces' its objects, the fact still remains that, after all the controversies, the sciences seem to have discovered a world that came into being without men and without sciences. Galileo may have constructed the phases of Venus, but once that construction was complete her phases appeared to have been 'always already present.' The fabricated fact has become the accomplished fact, the *fait accompli*. Diesel did not construct his engine any more than Galileo built his planet. Some will contend that the engine is out of Diesel's control as much as Venus was out of Galileo's; even so, no one would dare assert that the Diesel engine 'was always already there, even before it was discovered.' No one is a Platonist where technology is concerned—except for very primitive, basic gestures like the ones Leroi-Gourhan calls 'technological trends.' This rejection of Platonism gives greater freedom to the observer of machines than to the observer of facts. The big problems of realism and relativism do not bother him. He is free to study engineers who are creating fictions, since fiction, the projection of a state of technology from five or fifty years in the future to a time *T*, is part of their job. They invent a means of transportation that does not exist, paper passengers, opportunities that have to be created, places to be designed (often from scratch), component industries, technological revolutions." Bruno Latour, *Aramis, or The Love of Technology*, trans. Catherine Porter (Cambridge, MA: Harvard University Press, 1996), 23–24.

45. Jennifer K. Ladino, *Reclaiming Nostalgia: Longing for Nature in American Literature* (Charlottesville, VA: University of Virginia Press, 2012), 53.

46. Once again, the conflation of, quite specific, matter and, quite specific, symbol is deliberate. As Latour writes with reference to the study of technology or technological projects, more generally, "To study a technological project, one must constantly move from signs to things, and vice versa. . . . Depending on the point at which we look into the action, the 'meeting of the branches,' we will have ideas, drawings, lines in a program, trains running before our eyes, statistics, seductive stories, memories of trains running before the eyes of our interlocutors, photos, plans again, chips again. For the engineer substitutes for the signs he writes the things that he has mobilized; he attaches them to each other so they'll hold up; then he withdraws a little, delegating to another self, in the form of a chip, a sensor, or an automatic device, the task of watching over the connection. And this delegating allows him to withdraw even further—as if there were an object. If only we always went from signs to things! But we also go in the other direction; and we soon find ourselves not in a subway train but in a conference room, once again among signs speaking to humans—as if there were subjects!" Latour, *Aramis*, 80–81.

47. Pheng Cheah, *Spectral Nationality: Passages of Freedom from Kant to Postcolonial Literatures of Liberation* (New York: Columbia University Press, 2003), 382.

48. And also for problematizing it. Consider Braidotti's comment in her *The Posthuman*: "The feminist philosophies of sexual difference, through the spectrum of the critique of dominant masculinity, also stressed the ethno-centric nature of European claims to universalism. They advocated the need to open it up to the 'others within' in such a way as to re-locate diversity and multiple belongings to a

central position as a structural component of European subjectivity." Rosi Braidotti, *The Posthuman* (Cambridge: Polity Press, 2013), 25.

49. Rosi Braidotti, *Metamorphoses: Toward a Materialist Theory of Becoming* (Cambridge: Polity Press, 2002), 9. See also p. 36, on the problem of writing feminist theory in a context in which even "the feminine" might be "colonized by the male imaginary."

CHAPTER 1. FEMINIST THEORY AND THE POLITICS OF LIFE

1. Michel Foucault, *Society Must Be Defended*, trans. D. Macey (New York: Picador Press, 2003), 245.

2. Paul Rabinow and Nikolas Rose, "Biopower Today," *BioSocieties* 1 (2006): 195–217, 208.

3. Hannah Landecker, "Living Differently in Time: Plasticity, Temporality and Cellular Biotechnologies," *Culture Machine* 7 (2005), http://www.culturemachine. net/index.php/cm/article/viewArticle/26/33.

4. Braidotti, *Metamorphoses*, 242.

5. Foucault, *Society Must Be Defended*, 245.

6. For a review of some of this literature, see, Gabor Balazsi, Alexander van Oudenaarden, and James J. Collins, "Cellular Decision Making and Biological Noise: From Microbes to Mammals," *Cell* 144 (March 18, 2011): 910–925.

7. Ibid., 910–925; Dennis Bray, *Wetware: A Computer in Every Living Cell* (New Haven, CT: Yale University Press, 2009); Tanya Latty and Madeleine Beekman, "Irrational Decision-Making in an Amoeboid Organism: Transitivity and Context Dependent Preferences," *Proceedings of the Royal Society B* (2010): 1–6.

8. See chapter 2.

9. Lynn K. Nyhart and Scott Lidgard, "Individuals at the Center of Biology: Rudolf Leuckart's *Polymorphismus der Individuen* and the Ongoing Narrative of Parts and Wholes," *Journal of the History of Biology* 44 (2011): 373–443, 375.

10. Ibid., 379.

11. Ibid., 398.

12. Ibid.

13. Ibid., 398.

14. Elizabeth Grosz, *Becoming Undone: Darwinian Reflections on Life, Politics and Art* (Durham, NC: Duke University Press, 2011).

15. Although the executioner's hood does still fit when it comes to the classical philosopher-scientists and scientist-philosophers who floated Perfection in the first place.

16. Luciana Parisi, *Abstract Sex: Philosophy, Bio-Technology, and the Mutations of Desire* (London: Continuum, 2004), 49; Luciana Parisi, "Information Trading and Symbiotic Micropolitics," *Social Text* 22, no. 3 (Fall 2004): 24–49, 29.

17. Grosz, *Becoming Undone*, 27.

18. Ibid.

19. Ibid., 36. Eugene Thacker's discussion of Deleuze's complication of apparent boundaries separating the living from the nonliving (especially in the realm of living thought) is worth noting here as well: "Deleuze's understanding of Spinoza, and

of Spinoza's own pantheism, is uniquely indebted to the 'post-Scholastic' pantheism of [Nicholas of] Cusa. As Deleuze notes, 'The traditional couple of *explicatio* and *complicatio* historically reflects a vitalism never far from pantheism [*un vitalisme toujours proche du panthéisme*].' And, in this vein, what Spinoza accomplishes is to 'restore a Philosophy of Nature' to a place beyond the terms set out by Descartes. However, Deleuze is also careful to distance the pantheism of Cusa and Spinoza from 'vitalism' in its biologistic vein. If the processes of *complicatio* and *explicatio* are vitalist, this is because they have to do with the constant creation and innovation of forms, not because they teleologically lead to the animal, the organism, or the species, This is an important move, and it characterizes nearly all Deleuze's writing on Spinoza. This gesture—pulling vitalism away from biology and reconnecting it to pantheism—is also found in a more subtle way in Maurice de Gandillac's writing on Cusa. Gandillac, who was Deleuze's advisor for *Difference and Repetition*, also points to the inherently dynamic, processual qualities of *complicatio* and *explicatio*. Significantly, he also warns against an understanding of such processes that would reduce them to biology." Eugene Thacker, *After Life* (Chicago: University of Chicago Press, 2010), 209.

20. For a critique of this "transfer of blame," see Mark Francis, *Herbert Spencer and the Invention of Modern Life* (New York: Routledge, 2014), 295.

21. Grosz, *Becoming Undone*, 47.

22. Ibid.

23. Ibid.

24. Ibid., 69.

25. Ibid., 32.

26. Ibid.

27. Claire Colebrook, *Death of the PostHuman: Essays on Extinction*, vol. 1 (Ann Arbor: Open Humanities Press/University of Michigan Press, 2014); Claire Colebrook, *Sex after Life: Essays on Extinction*, vol. 2 (Ann Arbor: Open Humanities Press/University of Michigan Press, 2014).

28. Colebrook, *Death of the PostHuman*, 1:20.

29. Colebrook, *Sex after Life*, 2:11.

30. Colebrook, *Death of the PostHuman*, 1:21.

31. "If we are suffering from hyper-affective disorder this is because a potentiality of the body for undergoing stimulus but without conceptuality and attention is now no longer a background condition but accounts for the desiring structures of contemporary culture tout de court." Colebrook, *Death of the PostHuman*, 1:84.

32. Ibid., 1:21.

33. After all, consider Ketabgian's discussion of the piano in the Victorian industrial imagination: "this last chapter treats the industrialization of sensation and perception at another site and through another mechanism: the piano—or, to invoke its popular moniker, the 'musical steam engine.' As many Victorians viewed it during the century's middle decades, the piano belonged to the same realm as the factory and its machinery, and supported similar communities of mechanical habit and feeling. Blending musical passion with new standards of technical virtuosity, it promoted a variety of compensatory pleasures and practices, realized

through industrial rhythms, energies, and intensities. . . . Whether among listeners or performers, amateurs or professionals, the piano served both as a medium for intense spiritual affect and as a site of near-automatic technical skill—the ultimate complement to industrial habits and practices. *Marian Withers* especially stresses these dual aspects of musical technique, celebrating it as an aesthetic model of self-control while also warning against its penetrating, mesmeric influence upon the passions. Imagined as dynamic networks of minds, bodies, spirits, and forces, these technical communities stirred up a wide array of industrial fears and fantasies. Even for Karl Marx, the ideal 'virtuoso' was not a human but an industrial machine, 'which possesses skill and strength in place of the worker' and which realizes 'a soul of its own in the mechanical laws acting through it.' " Tamara Ketabgian, *The Lives of Machines: The Industrial Imaginary in Victorian Literature and Culture* (Ann Arbor: University of Michigan Press, 2011), 147–148.

34. Colebrook, *Death of the PostHuman*, 1:135.
35. Ibid., 1:136.
36. Ibid.
37. Ibid., 1:138.
38. Ibid., 1:139.
39. Dust is a key player in this show. At its first mention here, it's worth referencing Jussi Parikka's "Dust and Exhaustion: The Labor of Media Materialism," *C-Theory*, October 22, 2013, http://www.ctheory.net/articles.aspx?id=726. "Dust," he writes, "takes us—and our thinking—to different places and opens up multiple agendas. In this case, I use dust to talk of global labor, media materialism of digital culture, and how to approach this topic through such non-human nanoparticles." Or, alternatively, "dust, far from constituting the 'opposite thing to waste,' actually increases our understanding of waste as a process involving transformation and remainder, not erasure through expenditure. Even within electronics, which are guided by a sense of the apparent ease of dematerialization and erasure, it is possible to observe just how persistent remainder is." Gabrys, *Digital Rubbish*, 139.
40. Colebrook, *Sex after Life*, 2:136.
41. Ibid., 2:136.
42. Ibid., 2:248.
43. Ibid.
44. Ian Baucom, *Out of Place: Englishness, Empire, and the Locations of Identity* (Princeton, NJ: Princeton University Press, 1999), 51.
45. Paul Rabinow and Nikolas Rose, "Biopower Today," *BioSocieties* 1 (2006): 195–217, 208.
46. Bennett, *Vibrant Matter*, 23. Or, for a more evocative account—also more relevant to this study—see: "Scientists estimate that approximately ninety percent of the cells in the human body belong to non-human organisms, bacteria, fungi, and a whole bestiary of other organisms). Why shouldn't this also be the case for human thought as well? In a sense, this book is an exploration of this idea—that thought is not human. In a sense, the world-without-us is not to be found in a 'great beyond' that is exterior to the World (the world-for-us) or the Earth (the world-in-itself); rather, it is in the very fissures, lapses, or lacunae in the World and

the Earth. The Planet (the world-without-us) is, in the words of darkness mysticism, the 'dark intelligible abyss' that is paradoxically manifest as the World and the Earth." Eugene Thacker, *In the Dust of this Planet: Horror of Philosophy*, vol. 1 (Washington, DC: Zero Books, 2011), 7–8.

47. Balazsi et al., "Cellular Decision Making and Biological Noise," 911.

48. Ibid., 911.

49. Ibid.

50. Ibid.

51. Luce Irigaray, "The 'Mechanics' of Fluids," in *This Sex Which is Not One*, trans. Catherine Porter (Ithaca, NY: Cornell University Press, 1985), 106–119, 109.

52. Ibid., 111.

53. As Wendy Brown writes with reference to Adrienne Rich and Primo Levi, "Primo Levi makes drowning function as a symbol for a lost linguistic order that itself signifies a lost civil order, for being at sea in words that do not communicate and by which one cannot communicate. In a radically different context, Adrienne Rich also relates drowning to speech: "Your silence today is a pond where drowned things live." ... [W]hat if the accent marks were placed differently, so that silence becomes a place where drowned things *live*—a place where Levi's drowning inmates survive despite being overwhelmed by the words that fill and consume the air necessary for life? ... [W]hat if silence is a reprieve from drowning in words that do not communicate or confer recognition, that only bombard or drown." Wendy Brown, "Freedom's Silences," in *Edgework: Critical Essays on Knowledge and Politics* (Princeton, NJ: Princeton University Press, 2005), 93.

54. Rosi Braidotti, *Metamorphoses: Toward a Materialist Theory of Becoming* (Cambridge: Polity Press, 2002), 63.

55. Ibid.

56. Compare this approach to the operation of the brain as it is described by Alain Prochiantz in both Tobias Rees, "Being Neurologically Human Today: Life and Science and Adult Cerebral Plasticity (an Ethical Analysis)," *American Ethnologist* 37, no. 1 (2010): 150–166, 157; and Alain Prochiantz, *Machine-Esprit* (Paris: Éditions Odile Jacob, 2001), 38–39.

57. Braidotti, *Metamorphoses*, 63.

58. Ibid., 136.

59. Ibid., 228.

60. Braidotti, *Posthuman*, 193.

61. Parikka, *Anthrobscene*, 24.

62. Gary C. Cross, *Consumed Nostalgia: Memory in the Age of Fast Capitalism* (New York: Columbia University Press, 2015), 21.

63. Landecker, "Living Differently."

64. Ibid.

65. Ibid.

66. Ibid.

67. Ibid.

68. Myra J. Hird, "Feminist Engagements with Matter: *Judith Butler: Live Theory* by Vicki Kirby; *Psychosomatic: Feminism and the Neurological Body* by Elizabeth

A. Wilson; *Abstract Sex: Philosophy, Bio-technology, and the Mutations of Desire* by Luciana Parisi; *When Species Meet* by Donna Haraway; *Meeting the Universe Halfway: Quantum Physics and the Entanglement of Matter and Meaning* by Karen Barad," *Feminist Studies* 35, no. 2 (Summer 2009): 329–346, 343–344.

69. Luciana Parisi, *Abstract Sex: Philosophy, Bio-Technology, and the Mutations of Desire* (London: Continuum, 2004), 49.

70. Ibid., 56–57.

71. Ibid., 56–57.

CHAPTER 2. NONHUMAN NOSTALGIA

1. Braidotti, *Metamorphoses*, 41.

2. Ibid., 262.

3. Ibid.

4. S. D. Chrostowska, "Consumed by Nostalgia?," *SubStance* 39, no. 2 (122) (2010): 52–70, 53.

5. Ibid.

6. Ibid., 173.

7. Ibid., 64.

8. For a complementary approach, see "archivable data is calculable data. This is the other critical component of electronic memory: not only does it store, but it also programs material for operation. The computer is the universal machine. It can operate on anything as long as that material is rendered in digital format. The consequences of digitalization are seldom mentioned. While these electronic mechanisms may seem to preserve 'endangered things' in a relatively permanent archive, they also present the dilemma that . . . as we input heaps of data into digital devices, it seldom occurs to us that the digital devices themselves are rapidly changing entities and that they, too, generate data for the record. Moreover, the inability to archive itself means the electronic mechanism has a fundamental inattention to its own temporal configuration. When memory is apparently separated from material requirements, compressed as it is within a compact processor . . . [it] not only computes in much different ways but also variously comes to ruin. The electronic archive grows to prodigious proportions, yet this same archive may be completely inaccessible in less than a decade unless it is reformatted to keep pace with new electronic technologies. Ten thousand years may be ensconced in a six-foot cube, but without a means to access the data, we can only gaze wistfully at the minimal cube and wonder at the inaccessible 10,000 years that did, at one time, fire through its busy circuits." Gabrys, *Digital Rubbish*, 110–111.

9. Jean Baudrillard, *The System of Objects*, trans. James Benedict (New York: Verso, 1996).

10. Ibid., 14.

11. Ibid., 89.

12. Ibid., 41.

13. Ibid., 101.

14. See also "the move to archive 'everyday life' has led to the reinvention of the project of preservation, where almost everything constitutes possibly archivable material.

But in the attempt to archive everything, we would encounter the everyday and its 'distorted memories' all over again. With such all-encompassing means of archiving at our disposal, we are able to store everything, but in that ambitious documentation, we at the same time inevitably include the decay and oblivion that, at one time, it was the task of the archive to guard against. . . . The relevance of particular material as archiveworthy is less important within these systems than the ability to perform recall functions that suit the needs of the moment. The electronic archive does not, in fact, need to leave anything out." Gabrys, *Digital Rubbish*, 118–119.

15. Baudrillard, *The System of Objects*, 220.
16. Parikka, *Athrobscene*, 41.
17. Mark Crinson, "The Uses of Nostalgia: Stirling and Gowan's Preston Housing," *Journal of the Society of Architectural Historians* 65, no. 2 (June 2006): 216–237.
18. Ibid., 233.
19. Ibid.
20. Patrick H. Hutton, "Reconsiderations of the Idea of Nostalgia in Contemporary Historical Writing," *Historical Reflections* 39, no. 3 (Winter 2013): 1–9, 2.
21. Crinson, "The Uses of Nostalgia," 233.
22. Edith Wharton, Preface to *The Ghost Stories of Edith Wharton* (New York: Simon and Schuster, 1973), 9.
23. Illbruck, *Nostalgia*, 19.
24. Ibid., 22.
25. Ibid.
26. Ibid., 136.
27. Ibid.
28. Ibid.
29. Ibid., 179, 214.
30. Ibid., 250–251.
31. Boym, *The Future of Nostalgia*, 3.
32. Ibid., 11.
33. Ibid., 54.
34. This slippery, oozing city flies in the face of, say, Henri Lefebvre's dominated (or dominant) urban spaces: "Beginning with space-as-matter, paradigmatic contrasts proliferated: abundance versus barrenness, congeniality versus hostility, and so on. It was upon this primary stratum of space, so to speak, that agricultural and pasto ral activity laid down the earliest networks: *ur*-places and their natural indicators; blazes or way-markers with their initial duality of meaning (direction/orientation, symmetry/asymmetry). Later, absolute space—the space of religion—introduced the highly pertinent distinctions between speech and writing, between the prescribed and the forbidden, between accessible and reserved spaces, and between full and empty. Thus certain spaces were carved out of nature and made complete by being filled to saturation point with beings and symbols, while other spaces were withdrawn from nature only to be kept empty as a way of symbolizing a transcendent reality at once absent and present. The paradigm became more complex as new contrasts came into play: within/without, open/closed, movable/fixed. With the advent of historical space, places became much more diverse, contrasting much

more sharply with one another as they developed individual characteristics. City walls were the mark of a material and brutal separation far more potent than the formal polarities they embodied, such as curved-*versus* straight or open-*versus*-closed. This separation had more than one signification—and indeed implied more than any mere signification, in that the fortified towns held administrative sway over the surrounding countryside, which they protected and exploited at the same time (a common enough phenomenon, after all). Once diversified, places opposed, sometimes complemented, and sometimes resembled one another. They can thus be categorized or subjected to a grid on the basis of 'topias' (isotopies, heterotopias, Utopias, or in other words analogous places, contrasting places, and the places of what has no place, or no longer has a place—the absolute. The divine, or the possible). More importantly, such places can also be viewed in terms of the highly significant distinction between *dominated* spaces and *appropriated* spaces." Henri Lefebvre, *The Production of Space*, trans. Donald Nicholson-Smith (Oxford: Blackwell, [1974] 2005), 163–164.

35. Boym, *The Future of Nostalgia*, 251.

36. Ibid., 77.

37. For a variation on this theme, see "As more and more data flow through and into databases, something other than the logistical imagination is able to grow. Data mining allows for the identification of unforeseen relations and factors. Concentrations of data establish new centers of gravity as they couple with sorting systems, giving shape to an understanding and a politics based on probabilities . . . on the face of it, most databases are best understood as describing sets, operating through the working methods of predicate logic in that they allow the selection, differentiation, union, analysis, and possible projection of the attributes of a rela-tion . . . [but] a relational database is a topological machine. Any table of related data, a monograph or even a bus timetable, establishing links between a finite number of stable, discrete, and interconnected entities, constitutes a topological machine. They establish networks of relations, the points of intersection between data and what those data link to and trigger." Matthew Fuller and Andrew Goffey, *Evil Media* (Cambridge, MA: MIT Press, 2012), 116.

38. Boym, *The Future of Nostalgia*, 258.

39. Ibid., 354.

40. Or, "animal" in a more complicated way than we ordinarily find in popular Animal Studies works. As Tamara Ketabgian notes, the conventional anthropomorphizing bent in such literature is by no means a historical given. In the past, animals were as much mechanized as anthropomorphized: "According to received critical opinion, *Hard Times* supports life over the machine: it promotes animal spontaneity and 'vital human impulse' in their battle against the calculating and life-denying mech-anism of Coketown's 'hard philosophy.' Yet, if critics of *Hard Times* view animal impulse as rescuing us from the deadening grip of machinery, animals were also far more ambivalently colored in Dickens's period. Allied not with the higher faculties of humans, but with the rote operations or the machine, animal instinct emerged in any number of Victorian discourses as deranged, irrational, and potentially dan-gerous to the stability of civil society. At the heart of this web of metaphors is a

term that captures both the sentience and brutishness of factory mechanism: the *animal machine*. The concept is twofold: on the one hand, it envisions machines as bestial and instinctive organisms; on the other hand, it refers to animal bodies fueled by powerful mechanical drives that reproduce the hydraulic energetics of steam. Spanning a number of disciplines, this figure was commonly invoked by Victorian industrial critics, philosophers, and medical writers." Tamara Ketabgian, *The Lives of Machines: The Industrial Imaginary in Victorian Literature and Culture* (Ann Arbor: University of Michigan Press, 2011), 19.

41. Illbruck, *Nostalgia*, 42–43.
42. Boym, *The Future of Nostalgia*, 77.
43. Jeff Pruchnic and Kim Lacey, "The Future of Forgetting: Rhetoric, Memory, Affect," *Rhetoric Society Quarterly* 41, no. 5 (2011): 472–494, 475.
44. Ibid., 474.
45. Ibid., 477.
46. Ibid., 475.
47. Ibid., 482.
48. Ibid., 477.
49. Ibid., 487.
50. See also "Electronic time is fleeting. With this realization, we can dispense with narratives of enduring cultural records and instead begin to study this technology in its volatility. Here is a technology that would archive everything and even transform non-media into digital format. It can store this data with a silent and swift system collapse . . . the promise of absolute memory, of a record of everything, gives way to erasure. But . . . we can begin to uncover the temporal economy of these electronic memory technologies. Electronic archives depend as much on . . . transmission, it turns out, as on storage. Because the archive is more akin to a network than a storage shed, the archive is most effective when its contents translate into transmission, into the ready execution of programs. Memory, in this respect, always occurs as a kind of process does very little on its own. How many inaccessible hard drives from decades past can one stare at before realizing . . . [that] without a means of 'getting at the record' these electronic devices are little more than doorstops. . . . Electronics may have given us the nanosecond, but they have also given us digital decay. The latter is . . . less about placing ourselves on a known—even if imperceptible—timescale and much more about a set of unfolding temporal effects. Indeed, digital decay can be so disorienting that it may be difficult to gauge . . . whether the rubbish is in the past . . . or the future." Gabrys, *Digital Rubbish*, 112–113.
51. Luciana Parisi and Stamatia Portanova, "Soft Thought (in Architecture and Choreography)," *Computational Culture*, November 2011, 3, http://computationalculture.net/article/soft-thought.
52. Ibid.
53. Ibid., 10.
54. Ibid., 9.
55. A search on Google Scholar for "cellular decision making" returns 968 results.
56. Dennis Bray, *Wetware: A Computer in Every Living Cell* (New Haven, CT: Yale University Press, 2009).

57. Ibid., 225.
58. Ibid., 9–10.
59. Ibid., 142–143.
60. Ibid., 164–165.

CHAPTER 3. EMBRYOS

1. Florence Vienne, "Organic Molecules, Parasites, *Urthiere*: The Controversial Nature of Spermatic Animals," in *Reproduction, Race, and Gender in Philosophy and the Early Life Sciences*, ed. Suzanne Lettow (Albany: State University of New York Press, 2014), 45–64, 48. See also Jacques Roger, "From Reproduction to the Problem of Life," in *Buffon: A Life in Natural History*, trans. Leslie Pearce Williams (Ithaca, NY: Cornell University Press, 1997), 139.

2. Lee Alan Dugatkin, *Mr. Jefferson and the Giant Moose: Natural History in Early America* (Chicago: University of Chicago Press, 2009), 95.

3. Chantal Tatu, ed., *Emancipation, réforme, révolution: Hommage à Marita Gilli* (Paris: Presses Universitaires Franc-Comtoises, 2000), 236.

4. John Staller and Michael Carrasco, eds., *Pre-Columbian Foodways: Interdisciplinary Approaches to Food, Culture, and Markets in Ancient Mesoamerica* (London: Springer, 2010), 516.

5. Félix Hément, "Entretien sur la liberté de conscience," *Westminster Review* 134 (1890): 550, 550.

6. William P. Smotherman and Scott B. Robinson, eds., *The Behavior of the Fetus* (Caldwell, NJ: Telford Press, 1988), 44.

7. Georgette Legée, *Pierre Flourens, 1794–1867: Physiologiste et historien des sciences*, vol. 1 (Paris: F. Paillart, 1992), 27.

8. Joseph Altman and Shirley A. Bayer, *Development of the Human Spinal Cord: An Interpretation Based on Experimental Studies in Animals* (Oxford: Oxford University Press, 2001), vii.

9. Fatma Müge Göcek, *Denial of Violence: Ottoman Past, Turkish Present, and Collective Violence against the Armenians, 1789–2009* (Oxford: Oxford University Press, 2015), 225.

10. For a refutation of this slight on Darwin's originality, see Stephen Jay Gould, *An Urchin in the Storm: Essays about Books and Ideas* (New York: Norton, 1987), 51.

11. Georges-Louis Leclerc Buffon, *Oeuvres complètes de Buffon*, ed. J. L. de Lanessan (Paris: Larousse, 1884), 153.

12. Ibid., 207–208.

13. Ibid., 207.

14. Ibid.

15. Ibid., 207–208.

16. Ibid., 292.

17. Ibid., 296.

18. Ibid., 310–311.

19. Parisi and Portanova, "Soft Thought," 17.

20. Buffon, *Oeuvres complètes de Buffon*, 150.

21. Ibid., 153.

22. Ibid., 155.
23. Ibid., 155–156.
24. Ibid.
25. Ibid.
26. Ibid., 332–333.
27. Ibid., 157.
28. Ibid., 289–290.
29. Ibid.
30. Ibid., 290
31. Ibid., 158.
32. Ibid., 167.
33. Ibid., 325.
34. Ibid.
35. Ibid.
36. Despite Buffon's unusual eighteenth-century dismissal of the popular model of female reproductive passivity and male reproductive activity, however, it was *not* the seeming equality of sexual or reproductive behavior that leant to Buffon's work its significance to the study of gender. On the contrary, regardless of whether commentators and scientists worked on the assumption that males and females were equally active or on the assumption that males acted on passive females, *all* of their writing suggested that gender was the key determinant of what thought and life, what information and matter, would be stored, processed, and then disposed of. All of these writers made clear that, in the realm of reproduction, life, and thought, waste is a problem of gender. It is nice, in other words, to recognize that Buffon did not follow what is ordinarily viewed as the Aristotelian, male-centered model of reproduction—but this refusal to accept female reproductive passivity is not what lends to his work its relevance to nonhuman biopolitical democracy.
37. Vienne, "Organic Molecules, Parasites, *Urthiere*," 48–49.
38. Buffon, *Oeuvres complètes de Buffon*, 207–208.
39. For more on "how biological conception narratives recapitulate . . . gender stereotypes," see Franklin, *Dolly*, 42–43.
40. Buffon, *Oeuvres complètes de Buffon*, 238.
41. Ibid.
42. Ibid., 337.
43. J. B. Demangeon, *Anthropogénèse, ou, generation de l'homme, avec des vues de comparaison sur les reproductions des trios règnes de la nature* (Paris: Rouen Frères, 1829), 11–13, 105–106.
44. Ibid., 140–141.
45. Ibid., 11–13.
46. Ibid.
47. Ibid., 48–51.
48. Ibid., 48–51.
49. Ibid., 48–51.

50. Joseph François Louis Deschamps and Émile Flourens, *Cours sur la génération l'ovologie et l'embryologie fait au muséum d'histoire naturelle en 1836 par M. le Professeur Flourens* (Paris: Librairie Médicale de Trinquart, 1836), 95.

51. See, for example, L. S. Jacyna, "John Goodsir and the Making of Cellular Reality," *Journal of the History of Biology* 16, no. 1 (Spring 1983): 75–99, 81.

52. Deschamps and Flourens, *Cours sur la generation*, 179–180.

53. Jacyna, "John Goodsir and the Making of Cellular Reality," 81.

54. A. Aug. Duméril, *L'Évolution du foetus: Thèse présentée et soutenue à la Faculté de Médecine de Paris* (Paris: Imprimerie de Fain et Thunot, 1846), 157–158.

55. Hément, "Entretien sur la liberté de conscience," 8.

56. Ibid., 90.

57. Ibid., 89.

58. Ibid.

59. Ibid., 148.

60. Ibid.

61. William Thierry Preyer, *Physiologie spéciale de l'embryon: Recherches sur les phénomènes de la vie avant la naissance*, trans. (from German into French) E. Wiet (Paris: Félix Alcan, 1887), 18.

62. Ibid., 25–26.

63. Ibid., 52, italics in original.

64. Ibid., 434.

65. Ibid., 151, 169, 435, italics in original.

66. Ibid., 466–467.

67. Ibid., 475.

68. Ibid., 487–488.

69. Here, there is an interesting echo of Foucault's introduction to Ludwig Binswanger's *Dream and Existence*, trans. Forrest Williams (Atlantic Highlands, NJ: Humanities Press International, 1985, 1993), 51: "One cannot apply to the dream the classical dichotomies of immanence and transcendence, of subjectivity and objectivity. The transcendence of the dream world of which we spoke earlier cannot be defined in terms of objectivity, and it would be futile to reduce it, in the name of its 'subjectivity,' to a mystified form of immanence. In and by its transcendence the dream discloses the original movement by which existence, in its irreducible solitude, projects itself toward a world which constitutes itself is the setting of its history. The dream unveils, in its very principle, that ambiguity of the world which at one and the same time designates the existence projected into it and outlines itself objectively in experience. By breaking with the objectivity which fascinates waking consciousness and by reinstating the human subject in its radical freedom, the dream discloses paradoxically the movement of freedom toward the world, the point of origin from which freedom makes itself world. The cosmogony of the dream is the origination itself of existence. This movement of solitude and of originative responsibility is no doubt what Heraclitus meant by his famous phrase, '*idios kosmos*.'"

70. Charles Sedgwick Minot, *Human Embryology* (New York: Macmillan, 1897), 70.

71. Italics in the original.
72. Minot, *Human Embryology*, 79.
73. Bahaeddin Şakir, *Tıp Kanunu Dersleri* (Istanbul: Mekteb-i Tıbbiye-yi Askeriye Matbaası, 1908), 16.
74. Moreover, the tone of these passages is oddly similar to the tone Ernst Kantorowicz describes in the emergence of skeletons and cadavers medieval burial art: "It is usually said that the first to have himself represented as a cadaverous corpse was a physician of Charles VI, Guillaume de Harcigny, who died in 1393 and was buried in the episcopal chapel at Laon; in fact, not too much will be lost if we forget about the slightly earlier tomb of Francis I de La Sarraz, in La Sarraz (Canton of Vaud), the horrors of which would spoil the appetite even of an inveterate ghoul. There followed, within a decade after the Harcigny tomb, the now destroyed sepulchral monument, in Avignon, of Cardinal Lagrange, who died in 1402. The arrangement of this monument is complicated in many respects, and so is the reconstruction of details. One important feature of the composition, however, is indisputable: Lagrange was represented both as a naked, skeleton-like corpse and as a cardinal adorned with all the pomp and the regalia of his Dignitas. A slightly different type of tomb architecture, or perhaps only a more condensed and more dialectical version of Lagrange's monument, became famous in the early sixteenth century through the mausoleum tombs, at Brou, of Philibert II of Savoy and his Duchess Margaret of Austria, although here the horror of death was mitigated. . . . In all those cases, one is tempted to say with the poet: 'Of marble is the stone, and putrid there he lies.' We may think, though, of other words as well when contemplating those tombs of powerful princes spiritual and secular. For the decrepit and decaying body natural in the tomb, now separated from the awe-inspiring body politic above it, appears like an illustration of the doctrine expounded over and over again by mediaeval jurists: Tenens dignitatem est corruptibilis, DIGNITAS tamen member est, non moritur—"The incumbent of a Dignity may decay, the Dignity itself is nonetheless forever; it does not die." Ernst H. Kantorowicz, *The King's Two Bodies: A Study in Medieval Political Theology* (Princeton, NJ: Princeton University Press, [1957] 1997), 431–432, 435–436.
75. Şakir, *Tıp Kanunu Dersleri*, 99.
76. Ibid., 105.
77. Deborah Hauptmann and Warren Neidich, *Cognitive Architecture: From Biopolitics to Noopolitics. Architecture and Mind in the Age of Communication and Information* (Rotterdam, NL: Delft School of Design, 2013), 410.
78. Colebrook, *Sex after Life*, 2:246–247.
79. Gabrys, *Digital Rubbish*, 89.
80. Ibid., 120–121.
81. Ibid., 125.
82. Ibid., 67.
83. Ibid., 150.
84. See, for example, Erik Davis's discussion of William Gibson's use of Vodou as a trope in his early work. Erik Davis, *TechGnosis: Myth, Magic, and Mysticism in the Age of Information* (Berkeley, CA: North Atlantic Books, 2015).

CHAPTER 4. ALPHABETS

1. Pierre Rondot, "Trois essais de latinisation de l'alphabet kurde: Iraq, Syrie, U.R.S.S.," *Bulletin d'études orientales*, 5 (1935): 1–31; İsa Öztürk, *Harf devrimi ve sonuçları* (Istanbul: Adam Yayıncılık, 2004); G. Imart, "Le Mouvement de 'Latinisation' en U.R.S.S.," *Cahiers du monde russe et soviétique* 6, no. 2 (April-June 1965): 223–239; Christopher Looby, "Phonetics and Politics: Franklin's Alphabet as a Political Design," *Eighteenth-Century Studies* 18, no. 1 (Autumn 1984): 1–34; İlker Aytürk, "Attempts at Romanizing the Hebrew Script and Their Failure: Nationalism, Religion and Alphabet Reform in the Yishuv," *Middle Eastern Studies* 43, no. 4 (July 2007): 625–645; K. Mitsukuri, "The Intellectual Movement in Japan," *Science* 7, 172 (May 21, 1886): 450–453; Thomas G. Winner, "Problems of Alphabetic Reform among the Turkic Peoples of Soviet Central Asia, 1920-41," *Slavonic and East European Review* 31, no. 76 (December 1952): 133–147; Q. S. Tong, "Global Modernity and Linguistic Universality: The Invention of Modern Chinese Language," *Eighteenth-Century Studies* 43, no. 3 (Spring 2010): 325–339; Frank Billé, "Sounds and Scripts of Modernity: Language Ideologies and Practices in Contemporary Mongolia," *Inner Asia* 12, no. 2 (2010): 231–252; Nanette Gottleib, "The Romanji Movement in Japan," *Journal of the Royal Asiatic Society* 3, no. 20 (2010): 75–88; Mehmet Uzman, "Romanization in Uzbekistan Past and Present," *Journal of the Royal Asiatic Society* 3, no. 20 (2010): 49–60; Alan Sanders, "Mongolian Transliteration: From a Latin Alphabet to a Romanisation of Cyrillic," *Inner Asia* 15 (2013): 165–175; Charles Edwin Trevelyan, J. Prinsep, A. Tytler, and A. Duff, *The Application of the Roman Alphabet to All the Oriental Languages* (Calcutta: Serampore Press, 1834).

2. See, for example, the rhetoric of chains, links, and hops in "Government Report in Response to FISC Primary Order of July 9, 2009," August 20, 2009, http://fas.org/irp/agency/doj/fisa/fisc-081909.pdf, 58, pdf, 14.

3. Consider, for instance, the evocative title of Lewis's account of the Turkish language reform broadly, defined: "a catastrophic success."

4. Hale Yılmaz, "Learning to Read (Again): The Social Experiences of Turkey's 1928 Alphabet Reform," *International Journal of Middle East Studies* 43 (2011): 677–697, 677.

5. Birol Caymaz and Emmanuel Szurek, "La Révolution au pied de la lettre: L'Invention de 'l'alphabet turc," *European Journal of Turkish Studies* 6 (2007): para. 27, http://ejts.revues.org/1363.

6. Or, more accurately, within three months: "Dans un célèbre dialogue avec Mustafa Kemal, Falih Rıfkı [Atay] imagine une transition alphabétique graduelle, consistant à maintenir l'usage des deux alphabets dans les écoles et dans la presse pendant une période de dix à quinze ans. Mustafa Kemal répond: 'Au bout de 15 ans, il ne restera plus qu'une demi-colonne en alphabet arabe dans les journaux. Savez-vous ce qui arrivera? Que survienne une guerre, une crise, n'importe quoi, et voici que notre alphabet subira le même sort que celui d'Enver. Ou bien nous pouvons le faire en trois mois, ou bien nous ne le ferons jamais.' Cet échange de vues, devenu un classique de l'historiographie kémaliste, traduit le volontarisme performatif du régime. L'important ici n'est pas de faire le changement d'alphabet en trois mois mais de laisser entendre qu'on va le faire." Caymaz and Szurek, "La Révolution au pied de la lettre," para. 27.

7. Hüseyin Sarıkardeşoğlu, "Trafikde vasıta problemi, Tartışma," in *Türkiye'de Trafik Problemleri—Semineri (20-24 Şubat 1967)* (Istanbul: Sulhi Garan Matbaası varisleri koll., 1967), 196–198, 197.

8. Ibid.

9. Naşit Hakkı Uluğ, *Üç büyük devrim: Eğitim birleştirilmesi, şapka ve giyimin değiştirilmesi, Türk harflerinin kabulü* (Istanbul: Baha Matbaası, 1973), 177.

10. Boym, *The Future of Nostalgia*, 346.

11. Ibid., 346.

12. Sarıkardeşoğlu, "Trafikde vasıta problemi, Tartışma," 196–198, 197.

13. Öztekin Tosun, "tartışma," in *Türkiye'de*, 40; Mümtaz Çoruh, "tartışma" in *Türkiye'de*, 165; Cihanoğlu in *Türkiye'de*, 149.

14. De Leuw Cather International, Inc. *Updating of the Bosphorus Bridge and Connecting Highways Feasibility Study* (Chicago: Cather International, October 1968), 6–12.

15. Ibid., 10–18.

16. Ibid., 10–36.

17. I will address these exceptions in the conclusion to this chapter.

18. Geoffrey Lewis, *The Turkish Language Reform: A Catastrophic Success* (New York: Oxford University Press, 1999), 2–3.

19. İsa Öztürk, *Harf devrimi ve sonuçları* (Istanbul: Adam Yayıncılık, 2004), 36; Şekib in Hüseyin Yorulmaz, ed., *Tanzimat'tan Cumhuriyet'e Alfabe Tartışmaları* (Istanbul: Kitabevi, 1995), 311–312.

20. Lewis, *The Turkish Language Reform*, 27.

21. Negroponte, 1995, in Lewis, *The Turkish Language Reform*, 37.

22. Caymaz and Szurek, "La Révolution au pied de la lettre," paras. 20–21.

23. Hale Yılmaz, "Learning to Read (Again): The Social Experiences of Turkey's 1928 Alphabet Reform," *International Journal of Middle East Studies* 43 (2011): 677–697, 677.

24. Ibid., 680.

25. Ibid.

26. Ibid, 685.

27. Ibid.

28. See also "The biomass consists of tiny drops in which information is encoded within complex molecules being progressively recopied. Errors occur during this process. Most of them are eliminated from the biomass, the genetic memory, by very com plex devices. These errors are called 'unfeasible mutations'. A few errors escape those devices, and they constitute what is called 'biological evolution'. Although our optimistic ancestors (those who believed in progress) considered this evolutionary change to be positive because it allowed new information to be created within the biomass, from the point of view of memory it must be considered a serious drawback. It shows that the biomass is not a trustworthy memory: instead of preserving information it 'processes' it. This processing has implications for technical projects. Genetic engineering, which can be defined as the attempt to store acquired information within the biomass, must take into account that all information stored

there is subject to errors of transmission." Vilém Flusser, "On Memory (Electronic or Otherwise)," *Leonardo* 23, no. 4 (1990): 397–399, 397.

29. *İmlâ Lûgati* (Istanbul: Devlet Matbaası, 1928) [prepared by the Dil Encümeni], vi.

30. As Trix writes with reference to the Albanian alphabet reform, which influenced later Turkish policy: "I relate Sami Bey's proposal for a Latin-based alphabet for Albanian to his familiarity with the Latin-based 'Standard Alphabet' 25 of the German Egyptologist and linguist Richard Lepsius, a predecessor (1855, 1863) of the later International Phonetic Alphabet (1888). Sami Bey knew of Lepsius's work through his friendship with the Albanian linguist Konstantin Kristoforidhi, who had translated the New Testament (1872) into the northern Geg dialect using Lepsius's system. Lepsius's Standard Alphabet, which included more than 180 symbols and required the cutting of at least 200 typefaces, was designed to provide a systematic way to represent the phonology of any language of the world in European letters. It was totally impractical in that the extensive diacritics and unusual symbols were excessively expensive to print, but it was linguistically descriptive. Sami Bey adopted only some of the symbols from Lepsius, but Kristoforidhi's use of the Lepsius system for Albanian provided a high standard of linguistic fit of script with phonology, which Sami Bey followed in his subsequent Stamboul alphabet." Frances Trix, "The Stamboul Alphabet of Shemseddin Sami Bey: Precursor to Turkish Script Reform," *International Journal of Middle East Studies* 31 (1999): 255–272, 258. See also "As early as 1863, the Azeri playwright Ahunzade Mirza Fethali presented a proposal for a Latin orthography for Turkish,2 before the Cemiyet-i Ilmiye-i Osmaniye (Ottoman Society of Science) in Istanbul. A second event in Ottoman script reform, though less well known than Ahunzade's proposal, was the adoption by many former members of the Cemiyet-i Ilmiye-i Arnavudiye (Albanian Society of Science) in Istanbul, in 1879, of a Latin-based alphabet for Albanian. This 'Stamboul Alphabet' was designed by Shemseddin Sami Bey and, unlike Ahunzade's proposal, was immediately acted upon and subsequently adopted by the new Albanian presses in Bucharest and Sofia, from which it spread through southern and central Albanian lands, all still under Ottoman rule." Ibid., 255.

31. Ibid., 258.

32. Ibid.

33. For example, "he points out the desideratum in simple words, and lays down, as the first principle, that the *orthography of any language should never use the same letter for different sounds, nor different letters for the same sound.*" C. R. Lepsius, *Standard Alphabet for Reducing Unwritten Languages and Foreign Graphic Systems to a Uniform Orthography in European Letters* (London: Williams and Norgate, 1863), 31, italics in original.

34. "The *third* proposal was that of the author, and its object was only to bring the orthography hitherto used in science into more exact conformity with the laws of physiology, and to adapt it to practical purposes. The object of the meetings was rather to prepare the question for further discussion and examination, than to adopt resolutions which should be considered as binding. The physiological system

of phonology upon which the proposed alphabet had been based, was acknowl-
edged to be substantially sound." Ibid., 45.

35. "It has become possible to construct an alphabet, based on physiological principles,
answering all the requirements of linguistic science, and embracing all the sounds
contained in the two great alphabetical systems of Asia. This possibility alone justi-
fied, and indeed demanded, a new effort to reach the goal." Ibid., 39.

36. "The illiterate languages offer only the difficulty of determining the true pronun-
ciation of every sound without the important guide of an indigenous alphabet fixed
by the speaking people themselves. The sounds once being known, the signs are
easily applied." Ibid., 89.

37. "This third kind of life, the 'nameless thing' so often described by Lovecraft, is a
paradigm for the concept of life today. The concept of life encompasses so much,
from the most reductive biological viewpoint to the most open-ended ethical or
existential viewpoint. When definitions or criteria for life are given, even these are
subject to modification and revision. There is a sense in which the major problem
concerning life has to do not with its definition, and whether such a definition
is possible, but with the very *plasticity* of life, a shape-shifting quality exhibited
in all the different ways in which we use the concept to correlate to the different
phenomena that are deemed to be living—the plasticity of all the different ways in
which life is thought and shaped, all the myriad ways in which life reflects upon
itself and shapes itself, all the forms of existence, resistance, and insistence that life
is." Eugene Thacker, *After Life* (Chicago: University of Chicago Press, 2010), 3–4.

38. "It has been remarked above, that the general alphabet, when applied to particular
languages, must be capable of simplification as well as of enlargement." Lepsius,
Standard Alphabet, 79.

39. "With their capacity to disrupt the 'cold' automated linearity of formal languages,"
Parisi and Portanova write, digital accidents "encourage us to perceive a dimension
where algorithms have almost managed to 'come to life.'" Parisi and Portanova, "Soft
Thought," 2. In addition, "digital algorithms are autonomous, conceptual modes of
thinking, a thinking that is . . . a mode of feeling ordered in binary codes, and is
not to be confused with sensing or perceiving. Numerical processing is always a
feeling, a simultaneously physical and conceptual mode of feeling data, physical in
the actual operations of the hardware-software machine, conceptual in the grasp of
numbers as virtualities or potentials. Ibid., 4. Algorithms, in other words, "are not
only actions or pragmatic functions but also . . . suspensions of action or forms of
contemplation." Ibid., 17. When algorithms make mistakes, when they reach "the
limit of computation," they begin to *intuit*, rather than process, "infinite quantities
of data" and "incomputable information." Thus, algorithms are not only actions
or pragmatic functions but also, as Deleuze may call them, suspensions of action
or forms of contemplation of this infinity. These suspensions correspond to the
infinite discontinuities that algorithms encounter in the processing of binary unit
sequences, as these are always prehensions or captures of the incomputable data
haunting their own precise sequencing. It could be argued that these forms of contemplation may appear as glitches internal to the operational functions of the system. In fact, the conceptual prehension that algorithms have of infinite quantities

of data does not interrupt the digital operation but rather allows it to happen. In other words, whilst algorithms carry out the functions of processing, they are also conceptual prehensions of what lies at the limit of computation: an infinite amount of random (non-compressible) data. In this sense, algorithms are forms of contemplation, conceptual prehensions of incomputable information. It is important to point out again that such suspensions do not correspond to blockages but to the abstract passions of algorithmic thought, or the way in which ideas enter actual computational occasions." Ibid., 17.

40. Lepsius, *Standard Alphabet,* 175.
41. Ibid.
42. See also, for contrast, and the desire for total correspondence, "Johnson and his fellow-travelers encountered in the Highlands a landscape 'eloquent of its own history.' It spoke to them of a memory that spanned millennia and never failed, and of the standard of veracity to which their travel writing had to aspire. The language of lithic writing was a pure language, emphatically at one with its referent, and therefore invulnerable to that betrayal of meaning by expression which falsified human discourse. That natural language had the self-substantiating authority that was mimed by the quotations in the Dictionary—the English language's monuments to itself—as they shifted away from context and reference, and began representing only themselves, putting on the integrity and closure of a display mode at the same time that they put on the italic letter. The period's poetics of authenticity installed lithic writing on the same continuum of forms of representation that also linked the new notation systems inspired by tourism and the taste for ruins. These systems were those of lithography (literally, rock-writing), invented, one popularizer of that medium announced, 'to fix the free, original and rapid inspirations of the traveler who gives an account of his sensations'; those of the 'accurate delineator' and the 'camera-obscura.'" Deidre Lynch, "'Beating the Track of the Alphabet': Samuel Johnson, Tourism, and the ABCs of Modern Authority," *ELH* 57, no. 2 (Summer 1990): 357–405, 385–386.
43. Caymaz and Szurek, "La Révolution au pied de la lettre," para. 7.
44. Ibid.
45. Trix, "The Stamboul Alphabet of Shemseddin Sami Bey," 260.
46. "It is interesting to note that of the scripts historically used to reduce Albanian to writing, the Arabic script, enriched by additional symbols for the phonemes found in Indo-European Persian, required the fewest additional graphemes (seven); Greek required more graphemes (eleven), and the Roman script required the most additional graphemes of all (twelve) to represent Albanian. Obviously, simply phonemic representation was not the basis for the choice of the Roman over Greek or Arabic scripts." Ibid., 258.
47. Ibid., 260.
48. This claim rests on more extended work on "algorithmic politics" that it may be useful to explain here. The idea that both algorithms and politics are about doing rather than about expressing—about rules that define operations—underlies a great deal of historical and contemporary political thinking. The term, "algorithmic politics" might thus seem essentially redundant. The *numerical* quality of the

algorithm, however—the extent to which an algorithm is specifically a relationship among *numbers* that operate rather than among *numbers* that describe or express— has only recently begun to concern political theorists. As Shintaro Miyazaki writes, "while in algebraic notation a + b = c is merely a symbolic abstract statement which is not bound to any form of concrete execution, and thus can be changed into a = c − b or b = c − a. The execution of the assignment a + b ⇒ c is non revers- ible. Only once the values of a + b have been transferred and assigned to c can it get overwritten, reassigned to another variable or deleted." Shintaro Miyazaki, "Algorythmics: Understanding Microtemporality in Computational Cultures," *Computational Culture* 2 (2011): 3. It is this numerical quality of the algorithm that plays out across the Turkish alphabet reform. This brief introduction to algo- rithmic politics, therefore, will first, address algorithmic politics as a problem of *numbers*, and second, explore some of the implications of a numerically inflected variation on algorithmic politics. Miyazaki then continues, developing his idea of "Algo*rythmics*," that the Hindu-Arabic numeral system that became the basis for modern algorithms and modern computing differed significantly from the Greek and Roman numeral systems that influenced European mathematics throughout the medieval and early modern periods. Not only did the Greek and Roman sys- tems avoid the "concept of the number zero as a placeholder for powers of ten," but the "Greeks calculated mostly with shapes, lines, surfaces and things . . . not with numbers." Ibid., 9. As a result, "geometry," for the Greeks, "was more important than arithmetic," whereas in the Hindu-Arabic algorithmic system, "shifting, delet- ing, and adding positional numerals became the principle operations of calcula- tion." Ibid. Miyazaki continues by highlighting the materiality of this algorithmic mode of calculation, noting that "for a long time 'algorism' meant the specific step- by-step method of performing written elementary arithmetic inscribed on materi- als such as sand, wax and paper"—its "technicity" as opposed to its expressivity, and its relationship, again, to contemporary computing, where "the basic opera- tions . . . are still derived from the positional system not of ten states, but of two (0 or 1), which are then shifted, added, deleted and moved." Ibid., 2. In addition to privileging matter over space, that is to say, Hindu-Arabic mathematics, according to Miyazaki, also privileged operation over expression—symbols that do work over symbols that communicate. Following Miyazaki, algorithmic *politics*—derived as it must be from these Hindu-Arabic rather than Greek mathematical systems— might be best described as a politics concerned with symbols rather than with space. Moreover, the symbols that interest algorithmic politics are symbols that *operate* as they shift, appear, disappear, or move through, or as, matter. Material or spatial relationships that *become* numbers or that can be *expressed* in symbols are less important to algorithmic politics than numbers or symbols that are, them- selves, material. Numbers are not a handy way to express a more real or more true spatial universe. Instead, the operation of numbers, without space, and without expression, constitute the material universe. Algorithmic politics, therefore, is very specifically a politics of non-spatial and yet material environments given over to shifting, adding, and deleting. Functionality in these environments is numerical rather than spatial, operational rather than expressive or communicative. And indeed, as Miyazaki states, "a contemporary algo*rythmic* agencement"—in which "agencement" is "not only the network, but also all the actions that happen in the network"—"is still based on the timed and controlled sending, receiving, storing and processing of physical signals." Ibid., 8, 9. The algorithmic political "space" is thus never a space. It is a collection of actions and symbols, an environment of physical signals and numbers. Perhaps more provocatively, therefore, the key political figure within the algorithmic political structure, within the agencement that is simultaneously network, action, inaction, function, and dysfunction, becomes necessarily the algorithm itself.

49. Through the ostensibly useless labor that happens at the moment of the accident, therefore, through the seemingly meaningless doing and processing that characterize endless, accidental iteration, computational programs processing data are not only alive but political, reproductive, and biopolitical. Their productivity does not happen in aid of a specific, determined end, but as a mode of contemplation of the infinite. Their being and operation become, explicitly, for their own sake. Algorithmic politics thus assumes not only the algorithm as the key political figure, but an algorithm that exists, experiences, and thinks on its own terms. Or, as Parisi and Portanova emphasize, the algorithm is a symbolic operation that is neither a "subject thinking" nor a "thought object." "Soft Thought," 8. Drawing on the work of Whitehead, they show that numbers (like, here, letters) are not expressions of human thought, not symbolic tools that help humans or subjective minds work through mathematical problems, but, themselves, thinking machines: "symbolic operations . . . do the thinking for us." Ibid. Hence, symbols (numerical or alphabetic) in a computational or informational political context of the sort described by Parisi and Portanova are machines that both think and are thought. They are material modes of thinking that operate apart from any human subjective or syntactical communication or expression. The data set and the program that processes it, as a political activity, that is to say, feels, thinks, and acts unpredictably, by accident, while living in and through matter, and while producing an entirely symbolic physical world. Its life plays out in the accidents that move it either to zero or to infinity.

50. "It became necessary to discover a general system which might comprehend the two most important, but at the same time most widely separated, groups of the principal known languages. And it was evident that such a comprehensive system required a broader basis than any which had heretofore been proposed. That basis was to be discovered in the common ground from which both had started, namely, the *physiology of the human voice*, which is the common ground and standard, not only for the two above-mentioned groups of languages, but also for all the languages of the globe. The human voice has its natural bounds, beyond which no development of sounds is possible. Hence, the apparent infinitude of articulate sounds does not consist in a boundless extent, but rather in an endless divisibility, within assignable limits." Lepsius, *Standard Alphabet*, 38.

51. "La révolution de 1908 aboutit à la fondation d'une *İslah-ı Huruf Cemiyeti* (Association pour la réforme de l'alphabet) où domine le courant des *Hurûf-u Munfasılacılar* (les 'séparatistes'), qui proposent d'écrire l'ottoman en séparant

chaque signe, de sorte qu'à chaque lettre ne corresponde plus désormais qu'un seul caractère d'imprimerie. Pendant la Première Guerre mondiale, Enver Paşa, ministre de la Guerre, tente d'appliquer ce projet dans la correspondance militaire et de diffuser 'l'alphabet de l'armée' (Ordu Elifbası). Malgré son échec, c'est la dernière tentative sérieuse pour modifier l'alphabet arabe (Tekin 1984: 63–72)." Caymaz and Szurek, "La Révolution au pied de la lettre," para. 9.

52. "In the Constitutional period, the time between 1908 and 1919, those intellectuals who saw modification as essential were agreed that the letters must be written, or at least printed, separately, so that students and compositors alike might be spared having to deal with three or four forms for each letter." Lewis, *The Turkish Language Reform*, 28.

53. "The only scheme to be given a prolonged trial was the one sponsored by Enver Pasha from 1913 onwards, with the backing of his Ministry of War and, it is said, with strong-arm tactics to silence any critics. The principle was to use only the final forms of the letters, with no ligatures. The vowels were shown by variegated forms of *alif*, *waw*, and *ya*, written on the line with the consonants. The result was far from pretty. The system was variously known as *huruf-u munfasıla* (disjointed letters), *hatt-i cedid* (new writing), *Enverpaşa yazısı* (Enver Pasha writing), and *ordu elifbası* (Army alphabet). Originally intended to simplify the work of military telegraphists, its use was extended to official correspondence within the ministry." Lewis, *The Turkish Language Reform*, 29.

54. Or, as Parisi and Portanova put it in a different context, the matter "in and through" which the algorithm operates is neither "blind" ("Soft Thought," 9) nor "an extended software thought running on material bodies. . . .[Instead] we have a form of thought emerging from the iterative patterns and calculations of matter itself, suggesting a productive and constructivist notion of thought that does not describe but produces nature as it builds a constrained, ordered, objectified world. Calculation (or 'qualculation'), in short, is the way in which thought results from those material habituations (the repetitive algorithms) of matter, repetitive habits that allow all bodies to find their way or become oriented in space-time. Instead of an extended software thought running on material bodies, here we have a form of thought emerging from the iterative patterns and calculations of matter itself, suggesting a productive and constructivist notion of thought that does not describe but produces nature as it builds a constrained, ordered, objectified world. From this point of view, the linear causality of sequential algorithms shows that thinking is the same as tracing a grid in space-time." Parisi and Portanova, "Soft Thought," 12.

55. Or, consider N. Katherine Hayles's 2006 article on "the traumas of code," on the informational or computational accident as trauma, which resonates particularly well with this variation on living, reproductive, nonhuman, political memory. In this article, Hayles makes the case that code—and, in particular, the accidental code that does things "we have not consciously initiated"—acts as the "unconscious of language." N. Katherine Hayles, "Traumas of Code," *Critical Inquiry* 33, no. 1 (Autumn 2006): 136–157, 137. "Just as the unconscious surfaces through significant puns, slips, and metonymic splices," Hayles writes, "so the underlying code surfaces

at those moments when the program makes decisions we have not consciously initiated. This phenomenon suggests the following analogy: as the unconscious is to the conscious, so computer code is to language. I will risk pushing the analogy even further; in our computationally intensive culture, code is the unconscious of language." Ibid., 137. Starting with an analogy between the (human) psychoanalytic "unconscious" and machine code, and then drawing heavily on the extended mind model—"in which artifacts carry part of the cognitive load"—restricts Hayles's analysis to the realm of subjectivity studies. She writes, for example, that "[Nigel] Thrift's vision resonates with recent arguments for thinking of cognition as something that, far from being limited to the neocortex, occurs throughout the body and stretches beyond body boundaries into the environment. Andy Clark and Edwin Hutchins, among others, see human thought as taking place within extended cognitive systems in which artifacts carry part of the cognitive load, operating in flexible configurations in which are embedded human thoughts, actions, and memories. For Hutchins, an anthropologist, an extended cognitive system can be as simple as a geometric compass, pencil, and paper. It is not only a metaphor, he asserts, that drawing a line on a navigation chart constitutes remembering, and erasing it is forgetting. Clark carries the argument further to envision humans as natural-born cyborgs who have, since the dawn of the species, excelled in enrolling objects into their extended cognitive systems, from prehistoric cave paintings to the laptops, PDAs, and cell phones pervasive today." Ibid., 139. But if we bracket both the human touchstone and the extended mind framework that underlie her analysis, we can read her discussion of the trauma of code—of the digital accident as it relates specifically to *memory*—in a useful way. Hayles, for instance, argues first of all that trauma, like code, is "sensorimotor" rather than "linguistic," that it is "dissociated from language," and that it "resists narrative. . . . The characteristic symptoms of trauma—dissociation, flashbacks, reenactments, frighteningly vivid nightmares—suggest that traumatic memories are stored as sensorimotor experiences and strong emotions rather than as linguistic memory. Dissociated from language, trauma resists narrative. When traumatic events are brought into the linguistic realm, they are frequently divorced from appropriate affect." Ibid., 141. She continues that, indeed, the fact that trauma is "experienced consciously but remembered nonlinguistically" lends it "structural affinities with code": "Like code, it is linked with narrative without itself being narrative. Like code, it is somewhere other than on the linguistic surface, while having power to influence that surface. Like code, it is intimately related to somatic states below the level of consciousness." Ibid. Trauma, in other words, is according to Hayles one example of a distinctly computational, informational, nonhuman, and *physical and environmental* style of remembering. It is nonlinguistic and non-narrative—material, physical, and somatic rather than communicative. Here, though, perhaps more important than these qualities is the fact that traumatic memories are *accidental*. Their nonlinguistic, material quality is directly related to their ineffectiveness *as* memories. Or, put differently, they become functional when they cease to function—when contemplation and productivity do become the same thing. Like the embryo or the alphabetic character that becomes both alive and politically free at the moment that it encounters the incomprehensible—that begins to contemplate as it reaches the limits of processing—computational memory becomes contemplative when it turns into trauma (or nostalgia). When memories cannot be expressed but only felt, when memories cease to be symbols and instead become symptoms, that is when they are operational as memory, life, reproduction, and nostalgia. In short, the accident or the mistake lies at the heart of both the biopolitics of nonhuman reproduction and the biopolitics of nonhuman that this reproduction initiates. Or, more pointedly, the accident and the mistake that we see so frequently in politics broadly defined demand less explanation or remedy, and more the recognition that they are algorithms already at play. Indeed, as the ostensible problem of the alphabet reform demonstrates, politics already happens through matter and without space. It already involves symbolic operations that are both matter and machines—and symbolic operations that are both thinking and thought. It already assumes life and thought to happen at the moment of the glitch. And finally, it already has collapsed reproduction and contemplation. Moreover, the seeming illogic of memory in events like the alphabet reform ceases to be illogical when computational, embryonic, or simply nonhuman, rather than subjective, memory is the starting point. When memory is defined as something that involves program rather than content—indeed *forgetting* content in order to run programs—when it works through matter without space, and when it is contemplative only as it is uselessly, accidentally, and infinitely productive, then the problems that these seemingly contradictory memories pose to politics evaporate. These memories become not only internally consistent, but evidence of a functional, effective democratic biopolitics at work.

56. Lepsius, *Standard Alphabet*, 16–17.
57. Yılmaz, "Learning to Read (Again)," 679.
58. Caymaz and Szurek, "La Révolution au pied de la lettre," para. 41.
59. Ibid., paras. 20–21. Or, as Yılmaz also notes, "for someone fluent in French, such variations [between French and Turkish Latin-letter values] likely made generating Turkish in the new script a conscious, careful, and slow process, whereas writing Turkish in the Arabic script would have required no conscious thought and would have been comfortable and quick." Yılmaz, "Learning to Read (Again)," 691.
60. İmlâ Lûgati, vii.
61. Ibid., xiv.

CONCLUSION

1. See, for example, Devin Henry's thoughtful account of classical Greek approaches to the political problem of the embryo: Devin Henry, "Embryological Models in Ancient Philosophy," *Phronesis* 50, no. 1 (2005): 1–42, 3. Consider, also, the familiar—but also not familiar—difficulty that Aristotle, parsed here by Thacker, faced: "The *De Anima* is, then, an approach to this basic problematic: whether there can be an ontology of life that does not simply become either biological description or theological sublimation. And let us state up front the core of this problematic, which is this: Aristotle must presuppose that which he sets out to discover. In setting out to discover the principle of life, the 'is-ness' of life, Aristotle must presume

not only the category of substance, but, more importantly, the distinction between the living and the nonliving. The problem is deceptively simple. It goes something like this: Aristotle, in approaching the diversity of life forms, observes a set of characters unique to what he calls life. . . . These include life as defined by its forms (life as creative, inventive, and productive of different forms of life), life as defined by its temporality (life as characterized by movement, change, and alteration), and life as defined by a spiritual aspect (life as that incorporeal essence that remains the same; life as that immaterial essence that is common among all forms of life). In modern terminology, we might say that life for Aristotle is defined by form (life is the multiplicity of forms-of-life), by time (life is that which comes-to-be and passes-away), and by spirit (life is that which is common to all forms of life). In spite of—or because of—these characteristics, Aristotle is confronted with a challenge, which is to articulate a concept that is adequate to the diversity of what counts as 'life.' " Thacker, *After Life*, 10.

2. For an analysis of the problematic role of the embryo as person in recent French legislation, for example, see Bertrand Pulman, "The Issues Involved in Cloning: Sociology and Bioethics," *Revue française de sociologie* 48 (2007): 129–156, 130.

3. See also an interesting exploration of a different set of implications for such trash here: "a related kind of leak is not the accident but the elimination, the trash that takes itself out: insufficiently harsh deletions; waste dumps; secondhand trades in magnetic memory; tingles running through discarded hard drives; papers, due to be shredded or burned that make it as far as the dump and the freedom formed by decay . . . or by a pair of sharp eyes forming a gateway to the black market." Matthew Fuller and Andrew Goffey, *Evil Media* (Cambridge, MA: MIT Press, 2012), 101.

4. Chilea, "Le Régime juridique," 55.

5. Victoria Davion, "Coming Down to Earth on Cloning: An Ecofeminist Analysis of Homophobia in the Current Debate," *Hypatia* 21, no. 4 (Autumn 2006): 58–76.

6. As Braidotti writes, "parthenogenetic myths are always a sign of the potentially lethal powers of the undomesticated female . . . resurrect[ing] an ancient set of beliefs about the monstrousness of the female imagination." Braidotti, *Metamorphoses*, 196.

7. James Essinger, *Jacquard's Web: How a Hand-Loom Led to the Birth of the Information Age* (Oxford: Oxford University Press, 2004).

BIBLIOGRAPHY

Agamben, Giorgio. *Homo Sacer: Sovereign Power and Bare Life*. Translated by Daniel Heller-Roazen. Stanford, CA: Stanford University Press, 1995.

Agamben, Giorgio. *State of Exception*. Translated by Kevin Attell. Chicago: University of Chicago Press, 2005.

Altman, Joseph, and Shirley A. Bayer. *Development of the Human Spinal Cord: An Interpretation Based on Experimental Studies in Animals*. Oxford: Oxford University Press, 2001.

Aytürk, İlker. "Attempts at Romanizing the Hebrew Script and Their Failure: Nationalism, Religion and Alphabet Reform in the Yishuv." *Middle Eastern Studies* 43, no. 4 (July 2007): 625–645.

Balazsi, Gabor, Alexander van Oudenaarden, and James J. Collins. "Cellular Decision Making and Biological Noise: From Microbes to Mammals." *Cell* 144 (March 18, 2011): 910–925.

Baucom, Ian. *Out of Place: Englishness, Empire, and the Locations of Identity*. Princeton, NJ: Princeton University Press, 1999.

Baudrillard, Jean. *The System of Objects*. Translated by James Benedict. New York: Verso, 1996.

Bennett, Jane. *Vibrant Matter: A Political Ecology of Things*. Durham, NC: Duke University Press, 2010.

Billé, Frank. "Sounds and Scripts of Modernity: Language Ideologies and Practices in Contemporary Mongolia." *Inner Asia* 12, no. 2 (2010): 231–252.

Bonnett, Alaister. *The Geography of Nostalgia: Global and Local Perspectives on Modernity and Loss*. New York: Routledge, 2016.

Boyle, Eric W., ed. *National Museum of Health and Medicine: Guide to Collections*. Silver Spring, MD: Otis Historical Archives, 2014.

Boym, Svetlana. *The Future of Nostalgia*. New York: Basic Books, 2001.

Braidotti, Rosi. *Metamorphoses: Toward a Materialist Theory of Becoming*. Cambridge: Polity Press, 2002.

Braidotti, Rosi. *The Posthuman*. Cambridge: Polity Press, 2013.

Bray, Dennis. *Wetware: A Computer in Every Living Cell*. New Haven, CT: Yale University Press, 2009.

Brown, Wendy. "Freedom's Silences." In *Edgework: Critical Essays on Knowledge and Politics*, ed. Wendy Brown, 83–97. Princeton, NJ: Princeton University Press, 2005.

Buffon, Georges-Louis Leclerc. *Oeuvres complètes de Buffon*. Edited by J. L. de Lanessan. Paris: Larousse, 1884.

Caymaz, Birol, and Emmanuel Szurek. "La Révolution au pied de la lettre. L'Invention de 'l'alphabet turc.'" *European Journal of Turkish Studies* 6 (2007). http://ejts.revues.org/1363.

Cheah, Pheng. *Inhuman Conditions: On Cosmopolitanism and Human Rights*. Cambridge, MA: Harvard University Press, 2006.

Cheah, Pheng. *Spectral Nationality: Passages of Freedom from Kant to Postcolonial Literatures of Liberation*. New York: Columbia University Press, 2003.

Chilea, Dragoş. "Le Régime juridique de l'identité génétique de la personne en droit européen." *Curentul Juridic* 43 (2010): 53–68.

Chrostowska, S. D. "Consumed by Nostalgia?." *SubStance* 39, no. 2 (122) (2010): 52–70.

Colebrook, Claire. *Death of the PostHuman: Essays on Extinction*. Vol. 1. Ann Arbor: Open Humanities Press/University of Michigan Press, 2014.

Colebrook, Claire. *Sex after Life: Essays on Extinction*. Vol. 2. Ann Arbor: Open Humanities Press/University of Michigan Press, 2014.

Constable, Marianne. *Just Silences: The Limits and Possibilities of Modern Law*. Princeton, NJ: Princeton University Press, 2005.

Crinson, Mark. "The Uses of Nostalgia: Stirling and Gowan's Preston Housing." *Journal of the Society of Architectural Historians* 65, no. 2 (June 2006): 216–237.

Crockin, Susan L. "The 'Embryo' Wars: At the Epicenter of Science, Law, Religion, and Politics." *Family Law Quarterly* 39, no. 3 (Fall 2005): 599–663.

Cross, Gary C. *Consumed Nostalgia: Memory in the Age of Fast Capitalism*. New York: Columbia University Press, 2015.

Davion, Victoria. "Coming Down to Earth on Cloning: An Ecofeminist Analysis of Homophobia in the Current Debate." *Hypatia* 21, no. 4 (Autumn 2006): 58–76.

Davis, Erik. *TechGnosis: Myth, Magic, and Mysticism in the Age of Information*. Berkeley, CA: North Atlantic Books, 2015.

Delattre, G. A. *Traité pratique des accouchements des maladies des femmes et des enfants*. Brest: Imprimerie et Lithographie Roger et Fils, 1863.

De Leuw Cather International Inc. *Updating of the Bosphorus Bridge and Connecting Highways Feasibility Study*. Chicago: Cather International, Oct. 1968.

Demangeon, J. B. *Anthropogénèse, ou, generation de l'homme, avec des vues de comparaison sur les reproductions des trios règnes de la nature*. Paris: Rouen Frères, 1829.

Deschamps, Joseph François Louis, and Émile Flourens. *Cours sur la génération l'ovologie et l'embryologie fait au muséum d'histoire naturelle en 1836 par M. le Professeur Flourens*. Paris: Librairie Médicale de Trinquart, 1836.

Dugatkin, Lee Alan. *Mr. Jefferson and the Giant Moose: Natural History in Early America*. Chicago: University of Chicago Press, 2009.

Duméril, A. Aug. *L'Évolution du foetus: Thèse présentée et soutenue à la Faculté de Médecine de Paris*. Paris: Imprimerie de Fain et Thunot, 1846.

Essinger, James. *Jacquard's Web: How a Hand-Loom Led to the Birth of the Information Age*. Oxford: Oxford University Press, 2004.

Flusser, Vilém. "On Memory (Electronic or Otherwise)." *Leonardo* 23, no. 4 (1990): 397–399.

Foucault, Michel. Introduction to *Dream and Existence*, by Ludwig Binswanger, 31–80. Translated by Forrest Williams. Atlantic Highlands, NJ: Humanities Press International, (1985) 1993.

Foucault, Michel. *Society Must Be Defended*. Translated by D. Macey. New York: Picador Press, 2003.

Francis, Mark. *Herbert Spencer and the Invention of Modern Life*. New York: Routledge, 2014.

Franklin, Sarah. *Dolly Mixtures: The Remaking of Genealogy*. Durham, NC: Duke University Press, 2007.

Fuller, Matthew, and Andrew Goffey. *Evil Media*. Cambridge, MA: MIT Press, 2012.

Gabrys, Jennifer. *Digital Rubbish: A Natural History of Electronics*. Ann Arbor: University of Michigan Press, 2011.

Göcek, Fatma Müge. *Denial of Violence: Ottoman Past, Turkish Present, and Collective Violence against the Armenians, 1789–2009*. Oxford: Oxford University Press, 2015.

Gottlieb, Nanette. "The Romanji Movement in Japan." *Journal of the Royal Asiatic Society* 3, no. 20 (2010): 75–88.

Gould, Stephen Jay. *An Urchin in the Storm: Essays about Books and Ideas*. New York: Norton, 1987.

"Government Report in Response to FISC Primary Order of July 9, 2009." August 20, 2009. http://fas.org/irp/agency/doj/fisa/fisc-081909.pdf.

Greenwald, Glenn, and Ewan MacAskill. "Boundless Informant: The NSA's Secret Tool to Track Global Surveillance Data." *Guardian*, June 11, 2013. http://www.theguardian.com/world/2013/jun/08/nsa-boundless-informant-global-datamining.

Grosz, Elizabeth. *Becoming Undone: Darwinian Reflections on Life, Politics and Art*. Durham, NC: Duke University Press, 2011.

Hauptmann, Deborah, and Warren Neidich. *Cognitive Architecture: From Biopolitics to Noopolitics. Architecture and Mind in the Age of Communication and Information*. Rotterdam, NL: Delft School of Design, 2013.

Hayles, N. Katherine. "Traumas of Code." *Critical Inquiry* 33, no. 1 (Autumn 2006): 136–157.

Hément, Felix. "Entretien sur la liberté de conscience." *The Westminster Review* 134 (1890): 550.

Henry, Devin. "Embryological Models in Ancient Philosophy." *Phronesis* 50, no. 1 (2005): 1–42.

Hill, M. A. "Embryology." Blechschmidt Collection. https://embryology.med.unsw.edu.au/embryology/index.php/Blechschmidt_Collection.

Hill, M. A. "Embryology." Hubrecht Collection. https://embryology.med.unsw.edu.au/embryology/index.php/Hubrecht_Collection.

Hill, M. A. "Embryology." Kyoto Collection. https://embryology.med.unsw.edu.au/embryology/index.php/Kyoto_Collection.

Hird, Myra J. "Feminist Engagements with Matter: *Judith Butler: Live Theory* by Vicki Kirby; *Psychosomatic: Feminism and the Neurological Body* by Elizabeth A. Wilson; *Abstract Sex: Philosophy, Bio-technology, and the Mutations of Desire* by Luciana Parisi; *When Species Meet* by Donna Haraway; *Meeting the Universe Halfway: Quantum Physics and the Entanglement of Matter and Meaning* by Karen Barad." *Feminist Studies* 35, no. 2 (Summer 2009): 329–346.

Hopwood, Nick. "'Giving Body' to Embryos: Modeling, Mechanism, and the Microtome in Late Nineteenth-Century Anatomy." *Isis* 90, no. 3 (September 1999): 462–496.

Howlin, Patricia A., Tony Charman, and Mohammad Gaziuddin. *The Sage Handbook of Developmental Disorders.* London: Sage, 2011.

Hutton, Patrick H. "Reconsiderations of the Idea of Nostalgia in Contemporary Historical Writing." *Historical Reflections* 39, no. 3 (Winter 2013): 1–9.

Illbruck, Helmut. *Nostalgia: Origins and Ends of an Unenlightened Disease.* Evanston, IL: Northwestern University Press, 2012.

Imart, G. "Le Mouvement de 'Latinisation' en U.R.S.S." *Cahiers du Monde russe et soviétique* 6, no. 2 (April–June 1965): 223–239.

İmlâ Lûgati. İstanbul: Devlet Matbaası, 1928.

Irigaray, Luce. "The 'Mechanics' of Fluids." In *This Sex Which is Not One,* by Luce Irigaray, trans. Catherine Porter, 106–119. Ithaca, NY: Cornell University Press, 1985.

Jacyna, L. S. "John Goodsir and the Making of Cellular Reality." *Journal of the History of Biology* 16, no. 1 (Spring 1983): 75–99.

Kantorowicz, Ernst H. *The King's Two Bodies: A Study in Medieval Political Theology.* Princeton, NJ: Princeton University Press, (1957) 1997.

Ketabgian, Tamara. *The Lives of Machines: The Industrial Imaginary in Victorian Literature and Culture.* Ann Arbor: University of Michigan Press, 2011.

Kuhn, Thomas S. *The Structure of Scientific Revolutions.* Chicago: University of Chicago Press, (1962) 2012.

Ladino, Jennifer K. *Reclaiming Nostalgia: Longing for Nature in American Literature.* Charlottesville, VA: University of Virginia Press, 2012.

Landecker, Hannah. "Living Differently in Time: Plasticity, Temporality and Cellular Biotechnologies." *Culture Machine* 7 (2005). http://www.culturemachine.net/index.php/cm/article/viewArticle/26/33.

Latour, Bruno. *Aramis, or The Love of Technology.* Translated by Catherine Porter. Cambridge, MA: Harvard University Press, 1996.

Latour, Bruno. *Politics of Nature: How to Bring the Sciences into Democracy.* Translated by Catherine Porter. Cambridge, MA: Harvard University Press, 2004.

Latty, Tanya, and Madeleine Beekman. "Irrational Decision-Making in an Amoeboid Organism: Transitivity and Context Dependent Preferences." *Proceedings of the Royal Society B* 278, no. 1703 (2010): 1–6.

Lefebvre, Henri. *The Production of Space.* Translated by Donald Nicholson-Smith. Oxford: Blackwell, (1974) 2005.

Legée, Georgette. *Pierre Flourens, 1794–1867: Physiologiste et historien des sciences.* Vol. 1. Paris: F. Paillart, 1992.

Lepsius, C. R. *Standard Alphabet for Reducing Unwritten Languages and Foreign Graphic Systems to a Uniform Orthography in European Letters*. London: Williams and Norgate, 1863.

Lewis, Geoffrey. *The Turkish Language Reform: A Catastrophic Success*. New York: Oxford University Press, 1999.

Looby, Christopher. "Phonetics and Politics: Franklin's Alphabet as a Political Design." *Eighteenth-Century Studies* 18, no. 1 (Autumn 1984): 1–34.

Lynch, Deirdre. "'Beating the Track of the Alphabet': Samuel Johnson, Tourism, and the ABCs of Modern Authority." *ELH* 57, no. 2 (Summer 1990): 357–405.

Mbembe, Achille. "Necropolitics." Translated by Libby Meintjes. *Public Culture* 15, no. 1 (2003): 22.

Miller, Ruth. "Biopolitics." In *Oxford Handbook of Feminist Theory*, ed. Lisa Disch and Mary Hawkesworth, 61–78. Oxford: Oxford University Press, 2015.

Minot, Charles Sedgwick. *Human Embryology*. New York: Macmillan, 1897.

Mitsukuri, K. "The Intellectual Movement in Japan." *Science* 7, no. 172 (May 21, 1886): 450–453.

Miyazaki, Shintaro. "Algorythmics: Understanding Microtemporality in Computational Cultures." *Computational Culture* 2 (2011): 3.

Nyhart, Lynn K., and Scott Lidgard. "Individuals at the Center of Biology: Rudolf Leuckart's *Polymorphismus der Individuen* and the Ongoing Narrative of Parts and Wholes." *Journal of the History of Biology* 44 (2011): 373–443.

Öztürk, İsa. *Harf devrimi ve sonuçları*. Istanbul: Adam Yayıncılık, 2004.

Parikka, Jussi. *The Anthrobscene*. Minneapolis: University of Minnesota Press, 2014.

Parikka, Jussi. "Dust and Exhaustion: The Labor of Media Materialism." *C-Theory*, October 22, 2013. http://www.ctheory.net/articles.aspx?id=726.

Parisi, Luciana. *Abstract Sex: Philosophy, Bio-Technology, and the Mutations of Desire*. London: Continuum, 2004.

Parisi, Luciana. "Information Trading and Symbiotic Micropolitics." *Social Text* 22, no. 3 (Fall 2004): 24–49.

Parisi, Luciana, and Stamatia Portanova. "Soft Thought (in Architecture and Choreography)." *Computational Culture*, November 2011, 3. http://computationalculture.net/article/soft-thought.

Poole, Janet. *When the Future Disappears: The Modernist Imagination in Late Colonial Korea*. New York: Columbia University Press, 2014.

Preyer, William Thierry. *Physiologie spéciale de l'embryon: Recherches sur les phénomènes de la vie avant la naissance*. Translated from German into French by E. Wiet. Paris: Félix Alcan, 1887.

Prochiantz, Alain. *Machine-Esprit*. Paris: Éditions Odile Jacob, 2001.

Pruchnic, Jeff, and Kim Lacey. "The Future of Forgetting: Rhetoric, Memory, Affect." *Rhetoric Society Quarterly* 41, no. 5 (2011): 472–494.

Pulman, Bertrand. "The Issues Involved in Cloning: Sociology and Bioethics." *Revue française de sociologie* 48 (2007): 129–156.

Rabinow, Paul, and Nikolas Rose. "Biopower Today." *BioSocieties* 1 (2006): 195–217.

Rees, Tobias. "Being Neurologically Human Today: Life and Science and Adult Cerebral Plasticity (an Ethical Analysis)," *American Ethnologist* 37, no. 1 (2010): 150–166.

Roger, Jacques. "From Reproduction to the Problem of Life." In *Buffon: A Life in Natural History*, ed. L. Pearce Williams, trans. Leslie Pearce Williams, 132–150. Ithaca, NY: Cornell University Press, 1997.

Rondot, Pierre. "Trois essais de latinisation de l'alphabet kurde: Iraq, Syrie, U.R.S.S." *Bulletin d'études orientales* 5 (1935): 1–31.

Şaklı, Bahaeddin. *Tıp Kanunu Dersleri*. Istanbul: Mekteb-i Tıbbiye-yi Askeriye Matbaası, 1908.

Sanders, Alan. "Mongolian Transliteration: From a Latin Alphabet to a Romanisation of Cyrillic." *Inner Asia* 15 (2013): 165–175.

Sarıkardeşoğlu, Hüseyin. "Trafikde vasıta problemi, Tartışma." In *Türkiye'de Trafik Problemleri—Semineri (20–24 Şubat 1967)*, ed. Nejat Cihanoğlu, 196–198. Istanbul: Sulhi Garan Matbaası varisleri koll., 1967.

Smotherman, William P., and Scott B. Robinson, eds. *The Behavior of the Fetus*. Caldwell, NJ: Telford Press, 1988.

Staller, John, and Michael Carrasco, eds. *Pre-Columbian Foodways: Interdisciplinary Approaches to Food, Culture, and Markets in Ancient Mesoamerica*. London: Springer, 2010.

Tatu, Chantal, ed., *Emancipation, réforme, révolution: Hommage à Marita Gilli*. Paris: Presses Universitaires Franc-Comtoises, 2000.

Thacker, Eugene. *After Life*. Chicago: University of Chicago Press, 2010.

Thacker, Eugene. *In the Dust of This Planet: Horror of Philosophy*. Vol. 1. Washington, DC: Zero Books, 2011.

Tong, Q. S. "Global Modernity and Linguistic Universality: The Invention of Modern Chinese Language." *Eighteenth-Century Studies* 43, no. 3 (Spring 2010): 325–339.

Trevelyan, Charles Edwin, J. Prinsep, A. Tytler, and A. Duff. *The Application of the Roman Alphabet to All the Oriental Languages*. Calcutta: Serampore Press, 1834.

Trix, Frances. "The Stamboul Alphabet of Shemseddin Sami Bey: Precursor to Turkish Script Reform." *International Journal of Middle East Studies* 31 (1999): 255–272.

Uluğ, Naşit Hakkı. *Üç büyük devrim: eğitim birleştirilmesi, şapka ve giyimin değiştirilmesi, Türk harflerinin kabulü*. Istanbul: Baha Matbaası, 1973.

Uzman, Mehmet. "Romanization in Uzbekistan Past and Present." *Journal of the Royal Asiatic Society* 3, no. 20 (2010): 49–60.

Vatanoğlu-Lutz, Emine Elif. "Research on Embryos in Turkey with Ethical and Legal Aspects/Etik ve yasal açıdan Türkiye'de embryo üzerinde araştırmalar." *Journal of the Turkish-German Gynecological Association* 13 (2012): 191–195.

Vienne, Florence. "Organic Molecules, Parasites, *Urthiere*: The Controversial Nature of Spermatic Animals." In *Reproduction, Race, and Gender in Philosophy and the Early Life Sciences*, ed. Suzanne Lettow, 45–64. Albany: State University of New York Press, 2014.

Wharton, Edith. Preface to *The Ghost Stories of Edith Wharton*. New York: Simon and Schuster, 1973.

Winner, Thomas G. "Problems of Alphabetic Reform among the Turkic Peoples of Soviet Central Asia, 1920-41." *Slavonic and East European Review* 31, no. 76 (December 1952): 133–147.

Yılmaz, Hale. "Learning to Read (Again): The Social Experiences of Turkey's 1928 Alphabet Reform." *International Journal of Middle East Studies* 43 (2011): 677–697.

Yorulmaz, Hüseyin, ed. *Tanzimat'tan Cumhuriyet'e Alfabe Tartışmaları*. Istanbul: Kitabevi, 1995.

Žižek, Slavoj. *Absolute Recoil: Towards a New Foundation of Dialectical Materialism*. New York: Verso, 2014.

INDEX